Abdominal Pain

Abdominal Pain

Donald J. Currie, M.D., M. Sc.,
F.R.C.S.E., F.R.C.S.(C), D.S., F.A.C.S.
Associate Professor of Surgery
University of Toronto
Chief of General Surgery and Assistant Surgeon-in-Chief
St. Michael's Hospital

HEMISPHERE PUBLISHING CORPORATION
Washington New York London

McGRAW-HILL BOOK COMPANY
New York St. Louis San Francisco Auckland Bogotá
Düsseldorf Johannesburg London Madrid Mexico
Montreal New Delhi Panama Paris São Paulo
Singapore Sydney Tokyo Toronto

NOTICE
Medicine is an ever-changing science. As new research and clinical experience broaden our knowledge, changes in treatment and drug therapy are required. The editors and the publisher of this work have made every effort to ensure that the drug dosage schedules herein are accurate and in accord with the standards accepted at the time of publication. Readers are advised, however, to check the product information sheet included in the package of each drug they plan to administer to be certain that changes have not been made in the recommended dose or in the contraindications for administration. This recommendation is of particular importance in regard to new or infrequently used drugs.

ABDOMINAL PAIN

1 2 3 4 5 6 7 8 9 0 HDHD 7 8 3 2 1 0 9

Library of Congress Cataloging in Publication Data

Currie, Donald J
Abdominal pain.

Bibliography: p.
Includes index.
1. Abdomen–Diseases–Diagnosis. 2. Abdominal pain. I. Title. [DNLM: 1. Abdomen. 2. Pain. WI147 C976a]
RC944.C87 617'.55'075 78-31413
ISBN 0-07-014942-9

This book was set in Press Roman by Hemisphere Publishing Corporation. The editors were Rolfe W. Larson and Winfield Swanson; the production supervisor was Rebekah M. McKinney; and the typesetter was Ronald L. O'Dwyer.
Halliday Lithograph Corporation was printer and binder.

Contents

Preface

Little information is available on the origin and mechanisms of pain from the abdomen. Animal research on pain presents major difficulties, and there is a limit to experiments with human volunteers. Laparotomy under local anesthesia, the effects of interruption of sensory nerve pathways by local anesthetic agents and surgical operations, and sensory losses after various types of injury to the spinal cord provide information. Further understanding is derived from relating basic medical knowledge to symptoms and signs and by observing a number of patients with abdominal pain. The purpose of this book is to collect and correlate information that has been found helpful in understanding abdominal pain for all physicians who care for patients.

This book is divided into four main parts. The introductory section includes chapters on the embryology and innervation of the viscera and on the physiology of abdominal pain. The clinical investigation section includes chapters dealing with pain analysis and history taking, physical examination of the abdomen, and laboratory investigation. The next part covers clinical presentation and includes chapters on pain arising from various organs, diagnosis by pattern recognition, and systemic diseases with abdominal pain.

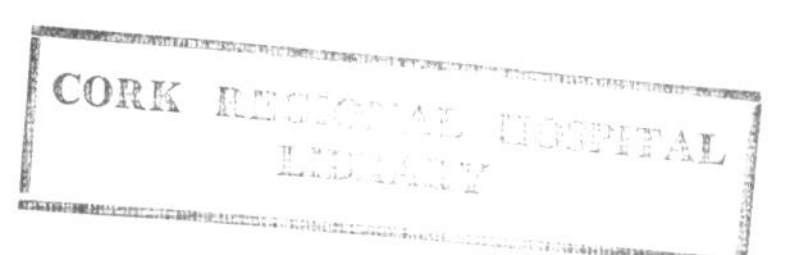

The last part includes the chapter on the principles of managing abdominal pain problems.

Some of my colleagues helped to revise the initial manuscript. All are members of the staff of the University of Toronto and, except for Drs. Diamant, El-Sharkawy, Orrego, and Taylor, all are on the staff at St. Michael's Hospital. I am most grateful to Drs. Nicholas D. Colapinto (general surgery) and Terrence L. Moore (gastroenterology) for reviewing the entire manuscript several times and for special help with a number of sections. Drs. Dennis W. Jirsch (general surgery), Edward J. Prokipchuk (gastroenterology), and Stuart Archibald (chief resident, general surgery) reviewed the entire manuscript. Because of his extensive assistance, I consider Dr. Ian Taylor (Department of Anatomy of the University of Toronto) coauthor of the second chapter. I thank the following people for special help: Dr. Donna Stewart (psychiatry), Dr. Hector Orrego, Dr. Nicholas E. Diamant, and Dr. Taher El-Sharkawy (physiology, gastroenterology), Dr. Robert A. Bear (nephrology), Dr. Bruce L. Bird (radiology), Professor A. Csima (biostatistics), Dr. Patrick J. Beirne (gynecology), Dr. Norman W. Struthers (urology), Dr. James P. Waddell (orthopedics), Dr. John K. Wilson (cardiology), Dr. James K. Yao (cardiovascular surgery), Dr. William J. Horsey (neurosurgery), Dr. Kenneth R. Butler (hematology), Dr. William E. Singer (endocrinology), and Dr. Randolph Lee (endocrinology, metabolism).

I thank Ms. Deborah Timmins-Jones for the early secretarial work and typing of the initial copies of the manuscript. My secretary, Ms. Jacqueline Bester, has performed all of the later work including the typing of the final manuscript. Mr. Harold H. Eckstein drew the illustrations. I appreciate the help of Ms. Anita Wong and her staff in the Health Sciences Library and Sister Pauline and her staff in the Medical Records Department at St. Michael's Hospital.

Donald J. Currie

Abdominal Pain

Chapter 1

Introduction

Pain is a disagreeable sensation resulting from unwanted irritation from the environment or from within the body. When pain arises from within the body, it is often unexpected, threatening, and unexplainable. The sufferer becomes a patient seeking explanation and relief.

What problems does the physician encounter in the physician-patient interaction when trying to help a patient in pain? What problems do patients have that make this interaction difficult? What is known about psychogenic pain? How does a physician arrive at a diagnosis? These are important topics for the diagnosis of abdominal pain.

Pain is the outstanding symptom of injury and disease and is the most frequent reason for a patient to seek medical aid. Pain demands the patient's attention and is a symptom feared by children and adults alike. In spite of its importance and frequency, little is understood of its nature. Acute severe pain demands prompt diagnosis so that immediate and correct treatment can reduce morbidity and mortality to a minimum.

Pain is not a pure sensation. Increasing heat and pressure eventually cause pain. However, there are receptors exclusive for pain that do not give rise to any sensation below the pain threshold. Generally pain is considered to be unpleasant and disagreeable. Occasionally, however, it can be sought by patients who gain pleasure from suffering. For these few individuals it may become a stimulus to bravery, a refuge, an excuse, a release, or simply an old habit.

The purpose of pain, teleologically, is the protection of the individual from external or internal injury. Without the protective nature of pain neuropathic joints degenerate, penetrating ulcers in insensible feet deepen, and infections in diabetics' feet progress. Superficial pain stimulates and exhilarates, preparing the person for action. Preparation for fight includes grimacing, frowning or closing the eyes, clenching the jaws, and tightening the fists. Preparation for flight may include crouching, flexing the limb joints, releasing or rejecting noxious objects, vomiting irritants, and running to mother. Visceral pain causes depression, withdrawal, and inactivity except when colic occurs. Nausea and vomiting are frequent accompaniments of visceral pain and tend to rest the gastrointestinal tract.

Pain is a personal, subjective experience. When a patient complains of pain, you have no choice but to accept this and seek the cause. Unusual attitudes and behavior may suggest a disturbed patient with psychogenic pain, but they may be part of the individual's reaction to organic pain. Never forget that mentally impaired patients can have painful organic disease despite atypical symptoms. An understanding of the clinical presentation of diseases associated with pain and the physical and psychological reactions to pain is needed to understand the patient's problem. Treatment can then be directed toward the cause rather than the relief of pain. However, it is correct to suppress pain when it no longer serves a useful function for either the patient or the physician. It is appropriate to provide adequate analgesia for early relief of pain when the cause is transient and unimportant or uncontrollable as in terminal malignant disease.

THREE ATTRIBUTES OF PAIN

There are three major responses of an individual: the intellectual, the physical, and the emotional. The equivalent attributes of pain involve the perception of pain and the physiological and psychological reactions to pain (Figure 1).

Perception of Pain

Perception of pain is the conscious or subjective experience of feeling pain. This perception is probably similar for most people. It is probable that the same intensity of stimulation gives the same amount of pain to all people, that specific areas of the body have similar sensitivity in all people, and that everyone has the same threshold for pain (53).

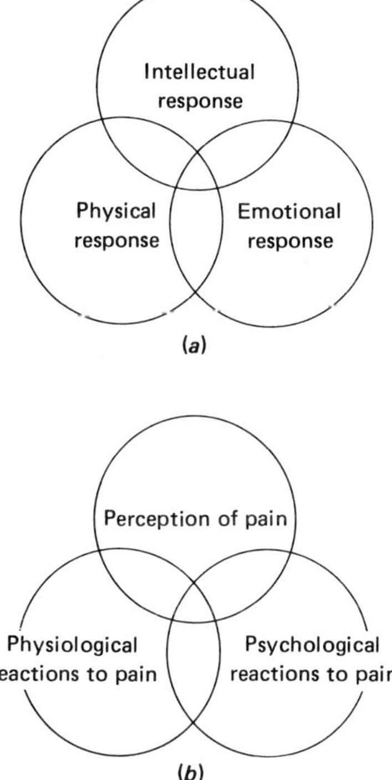

Figure 1 The three general responses (*a*) and the corresponding attributes of pain (*b*).

Nerve pathways for the perception of pain must be intact. This includes a living end structure, intact afferent nerves without analgesic blockage, and a receptive central nervous system. Exceptions are central pain, which has no peripheral representation, and instances where the peripheral representation is lost or damaged as in phantom limb pain and causalgia. Psychogenic pain appears to arise in the mind as no peripheral cause can be found.

The dimensions of pain include quality, intensity, extent, and temporal factors. The quality of pain sensation is resolved into two types; superficial pain is a prick, burning, or throbbing sensation whereas visceral pain is a steady aching or an intermittent colic (32). Intensity varies from threshold to maximal—the more intense the stimulation the more intense the sensation. The extent of pain refers to its site, location, and area. Temporal factors include duration, frequency, rhythm, and periodicity.

Physiological Reactions to Pain

The physiological reactions involve neural reflexes mediated through the autonomic nervous system. These reactions also involve reflexes that prepare the body for flight or fight when external stimuli cause pain or for withdrawal and immobility when internal stimuli cause pain.

The pain experience produces reactions both dependent on and independent of the state of consciousness. The physiological reactions are independent of the state of consciousness. There may be minor or major tissue damage at the site of stimulation or no perceptible damage to tissues. The reflex reactions are mediated chiefly by the autonomic nervous system and include pilomotor and smooth muscle contraction, involuntary skeletal muscle contraction, tachycardia, hypertension, perspiration, release of adrenal hormones and vasoactive polypeptides, and hypothalamic neural transmitter stimulation. The threshold for pain diminishes locally and central excitation occurs. The physiology of pain is discussed in Chapter 3.

Psychological Reactions to Pain

Psychological reactions, the major component in suffering, vary greatly depending upon many factors. Fear and anxiety may accompany pain and discomfort and may be followed by sadness, self-pity, and depression. Such reactions vary according to the patient's personality and mood. Psychological reactions to pain include changes in mood, attitudes, and behavior. These changes may be modified by conditioning, past experience, or cultural development. Other factors that alter these reactions include drugs, distraction, suggestion, hypnosis, environmental setting, and altered brain function. The psychology of pain is discussed below.

The three responses to pain have an important bearing on the management of individuals having pain. In treating these patients all three reactions must be considered. In cases of acute severe pain there is no doubt that the perception of pain needs prime attention. Strong analgesia is most important; usually narcotics are required. When pain is more prolonged, psychological reactions often become more important than the sensation of pain itself.

SOURCES OF INFORMATION

Because pain sensation is subjective, animal experimentation can help little in investigation. The nerve pathways for pain have been traced in animals by observing microscopic nerve fiber disappearance after nerve sectioning. Although it is impossible to measure pain in the experimental animal, it is possible to assess some of the accompanying reactions; pain relief poses similar measurement problems.

Most of our information comes from human experiment and experience, especially from study of nerve pathways and the patterns of referred pain. Relief of pain by nerve block or by local anesthetic agents confirms the route of pain impulses. During operations performed under local anesthesia, unanesthetized parts can be stimulated. The effects of nerve resection such as sympathectomy, vagotomy, and presacral neurectomy on the sensation of pain are revealing. Paraplegics and quadriplegics have been studied, and the sensibility of various internal organs has been related to the level of spinal cord injury. Sensitivity of the mucous membrane can be studied in patients having fistulae and intestinal stomata. Human volunteers have swallowed ballooned tubes and have reported pain as the balloons are distended at various levels in the gastrointestinal tract. Correlation of embryology, anatomy, physiology, and pathology with clinical experience has contributed much to our knowledge of pain sensation in the abdomen, pelvis, and chest.

HISTORICAL NOTE ON PAIN FROM DEEP STRUCTURES

Viscera have long been noted to be insensitive to most of the stimuli that evoke pain when applied to the skin. Toward the end of the last century abdominal operations were performed under local anesthesia, and careful observers found that pain could arise from the viscera and the walls of the body cavities. In 1888 Ross (43) was one of the first to record that there were two types of pain arising from the abdomen. He described visceral, or splanchnic, pain, which he thought was felt in the general region of the organ stimulated, and somatic, or parietal, pain, which he said was felt in the abdominal or chest wall.

In 1893 Head (16) systematically mapped areas of cutaneous hyperalgesia corresponding to the sites of referred pain in diseases of various viscera. He showed that these areas were in the same spinal segment as the nerves supplying the diseased organ. These areas are known as the Head zones of cutaneous hyperalgesia.

In the same year Mackenzie (35) disputed Ross's concept of visceral pain and suggested that all pain of visceral disease was felt in the body wall. Insensitive impulses from the viscera set up an irritable focus in the spinal cord so that sensations from somatic afferent nerves in that segment were potentiated, leading to pain impulses in the secondary afferent neurons of the spinal cord. The irritable focus potentiated spinal cord reflexes giving rise to muscle guarding, hyperalgesia, hyperesthesia, and tenderness. The brain would presumably interpret the pain as coming from another branch of the same somatic afferent nerve. This was called the viscerosensory reflex theory, and it was widely held for many years despite the objections of Ross and Head (36).

Lennander (29-31) is given credit for the first recording in medical literature (1901) that cutting, burning, or crushing bowel did not cause pain in the conscious subject during abdominal operations performed under local anesthesia. The only way pain could be elicited from the bowel was by traction on its mesentery, stimulating posterior parietal peritoneum. In cases of colic Lennander supposed that the powerful contractions of the gut put tension on the mesentery and so produced pain mechanically.

In 1911 Hertz (18) found that visceral pain could arise from nerve endings in the wall of the gut by an increase in tension. In 1948 Kinsella (25) wrote that the adequate stimulus for visceral pain was compression of nerve fibers in the bowel wall. Squeezing an inflamed appendix was painful, and he proposed that inflammation increases the sensitivity of viscera to painful stimuli. Wolff and Wolf (53) found that inflamed gastric mucosa was sensitive, but normal gastric mucosa was insensitive.

Morley (38), using acute appendicitis as an example, wrote in 1928 that direct visceral sensation did exist and that referred pain occurred only when inflammation reached the parietal peritoneum nearest the diseased viscus. His theory, often called the peritoneocutaneous reflex theory, does not explain referred pain in the absence of inflammation.

Lewis (32) showed in 1942 that subjects can distinguish only two qualities of pain, that arising from the skin and that arising from structures deep to the skin. If the skin is stimulated, a sudden prick or a more prolonged burning sensation occurs. If deeper structures only are stimulated, then a vague aching occurs. This indicated that the quality of pain as described by patients did not help in differentiating one pain from another but did help the physician to decide whether the pain was superficial, somatic, or visceral.

In 1931 Polland and Bloomfield (40) and in 1938 Jones (21, 22) produced visceral pain in human volunteers by distending balloons at various levels in the gastrointestinal tract. They showed that distension rather than other stimuli such as cutting, pinching, or burning is adequate stimulus for visceral pain. In 1930 White (51) used sympathetic nerve blocks to confirm pain pathways and predict the effects of sympathectomy.

In 1939 Kellgren (24) made important contributions to the localization of pain by showing that the referral of pain from somatic structures follows a segmental pattern. Pain arising from nonvisceral structures might have exactly the same area of distribution as pain arising from viscera. Deep tenderness and muscle contraction arising from irritation of a deep structure could be indistinguishable from that arising from a visceral lesion.

Wolff and Wolf (53) pointed out in 1948 that visceral pain can be referred segmentally like deep pain. They suggested that spread of excitation in the spinal cord, a central excitory state, accounts for the brain's interpreting visceral pain as coming from another peripheral branch of the same spinal nerve. They found that if hyperalgesia occurs at the site of a referred pain, then the referred pain phenomenon can be abolished by infiltration of a local anesthetic agent into the site of hyperalgesia. They also suggested that the spread of excitation can cause skeletal muscle contraction that can cause pain, and this pain may be abolished by infiltration of a local anesthetic agent into the contracted muscle.

Because there are more primary afferent neurons in the peripheral nerves than secondary afferent neurons in the spinal cord, Ruch (44) suggested in 1965 that both visceral and somatic afferents probably converge on the same secondary neurons. The brain, conditioned by previous experience, may then interpret the incoming visceral pain as coming from the skin. In 1965 Melzak and Wall (37) suggested that a presynaptic filter is set by supraspinal activity or by an afferent barrage of preceding sensation, and pain is appreciated only when the sum total of all afferent impulses exceeds a preset level. The gate control theory has special importance in the management of chronic pain syndromes and in understanding counterirritants including acupuncture.

In summary the viscera are insensitive to sensations other than pain and to stimuli other than increase in tension and ischemia. The root of the mesentery and the parietal peritoneum are sensitive to the same stimuli as the skin. Referred pain can arise with deep pain and even with visceral pain if sufficiently severe. Inflammation increases the sensibility of all sensitive parts of the body. Deep pain, either visceral or somatic, may be accompanied by referred pain, hyperalgesia, hyperesthesia, and sustained muscle contraction. These phenomena generally remain within the segmental or dermatomal level of the original stimulation, although spread can occur to adjacent segments, most often in a cephalad direction.

TYPES OF PAIN

Referring only to the quality of pain, superficial and visceral pain are the only two types. Deep pain is a mixed type having some of the qualities of both superficial and visceral pain.

Superficial Pain

Superficial pain arises from stimulation of the surface of the body by external stimuli. Such stimuli cause clear, sharp, acute pain, well localized, and generally familiar or easily explained. Superficial pain is carried in cutaneous sensory branches of the cranial and spinal nerves. Superficial pain warns of an environmental threat and is appreciated as the most common sensation resulting from injury. Superficial pain alerts and prepares for fight or flight.

Deep Pain

Visceral Pain

Visceral pain is the only type of pain that arises exclusively from internal viscera. It is either a dull, aching steady pain or an intermittent colic. Most patients find it unfamiliar and unexplainable. When visceral pain is severe, it may be associated with referred pain, reflex muscle contraction, hyperalgesia, and hyperesthesia. Visceral pain is a warning of a threat from within the body and is appreciated as the prime sensation of internal disease. Abdominal visceral pain is carried in visceral sensory branches of the vagus nerve and most of the spinal nerves. Visceral pain warns the individual of illness and leads to immobility and withdrawal. Visceral pain is also called splanchnic pain.

Nonvisceral Pain

Nonvisceral pain arises from internal parts of the body other than viscera and is stimulated by disease or injury. The quality of the pain is a mixture of clear, well-localized sharp pain similar to superficial pain, and dull, aching steady pain similar to steady visceral pain. Colic arises only from hollow viscera and is therefore not part of nonvisceral deep pain. Nonvisceral deep pain may be unfamiliar and unexplainable. It is a warning of changes within the body. Deep pain may arise from joints, ligaments, tendons, muscles, nerves, blood vessels, and the lining of the walls of the body cavities. Deep pain arising from musculoskeletal structures, nerves, and blood vessels is often called somatic pain. Deep pain arising from the lining of the walls of body cavities is often called parietal pain. The site of the pain is clearly localized but not as precisely as superficial pain. Deep pain is carried in somatic sensory branches of the cranial and spinal nerves.

PHENOMENA ASSOCIATED WITH DEEP PAIN

Referred pain is a pain felt in a region of the body other than the site of stimulation. The more intense the stimulation, the more likely referred pain is to occur, and generally the greater is the area of reference (53). Referred pain generally follows the rule of segmental distribution, which means that referred pain appears in an area of the body supplied by afferent nerves of the same spinal segment as the afferent nerves carrying the original stimulus. There may be overlapping or nearby spread of the referred pain to an adjacent segment or, rarely, two. This spread tends to occur in a cranial rather than in a caudal direction. Very rarely spread occurs to the same segment on the opposite side of the body.

Reflex muscle contraction occurs in association with nonvisceral deep pain whether somatic or parietal and also with severe visceral pain. It is segmental, centered on the segment receiving the original stimulus, and usually involves a muscle group. When the original stimulus is intense it often involves all of the muscles of that region, including the muscles on both sides of the body. Muscle guarding of the flat muscles of the abdominal wall is typical of the muscle contraction associated with deep pain. Involuntary muscle guarding, splinting, and boardlike rigidity are examples of involuntary muscle contraction associated with severe deep pain. Sustained muscle contraction causes pain, muscle tenderness, and a feeling of tightness in the region. In the thorax or upper abdominal regions the patient feels a tight restriction to respiration with a smothering feeling as if there were pressure on the chest.

Hyperalgesia is an excessive sensibility to pain and is another reflex phenomenon that occurs with severe pain. It may be caused by lowering of the pain threshold as occurs with inflamed, hyperemic, or damaged tissues where pain perception is more acute and severe and is accompanied by local tenderness. Hyperalgesia follows segmental distribution quite closely.

Hyperesthesia is excessive sensibility of a part, not necessarily to pain. This excessive sensibility also follows segmental distribution and is usually associated with hyperalgesia.

PSYCHOLOGY OF PAIN

There are a number of factors that influence an individual's awareness of the sensation of pain.

The *pain threshold* is the minimal stimulus for its perception and is believed to be the same for all persons (3, 15), although the physiological and psychological reactions differ greatly. Perception threshold may be raised by distraction, suggestion, hypnosis, or extinction. Drugs that can be used to raise the pain threshold include analgesics and epinephrine, occasionally given to soldiers and athletes. Pain threshold may be lowered by apprehension, anticipation, repetition, inflammation, or local tissue damage.

Alertness has a direct bearing on the awareness of pain. The hyperexcited person may overreact to pain. The more alert the subject, the clearer is the perception of pain. The semiconscious individual may react to pain after other sensory perceptions are lost. The unconscious patient may show no evidence of pain perception other than certain autonomic reflex reactions. In deep coma and under full general anesthesia even these reactions may be lost. Similarly deep or visceral pain below the level of injury in a paraplegic or quadriplegic are not felt, but there may be nausea, a feeling of being unwell, flushing, or palpitations.

Training and upbringing influence reactions to pain. Individuals may be taught to bear pain without showing it. If a person is taught to accept pain, voluntary muscle responses can be suppressed. If the psychological reaction to pain is condoned, the reaction may be excessively violent emotionally. For some individuals pain is a thing to be hidden and regarded as a sign of weakness, whereas for others it can claim special attention and be a cause for demonstration. For some it is a threat to be relieved at once, for others a suffering to be bravely endured. It may be a way of life or an intrusion. Individuals' reactions may reflect their training rather than spontaneous responses.

Past experience or previous events influence reactions to pain. Although the first exposure may be borne stoically, repeated exposures may not be borne as well, as the individual becomes fearful from anticipation of the return of the disagreeable experience. With repeated exposures and increasing resignation or fortitude reactions to pain may diminish or disappear entirely. Pain arising in structures rarely stimulated may be misinterpreted as coming from a structure innervated by the same spinal nerve but commonly stimulated. Lack of previous experience with pain in the prime area leads to misinterpretation.

The psychological reaction to pain varies widely with different *social and cultural customs.* In some cultures stoicism and self-control are virtues, whereas in others demonstration of painful experiences is accepted and approved. Some believe pain has health and medical implications, whereas others imbue it with magical and religious connotations.

Knowledge, understanding, and familiarity of the origin of pain influence reactions to pain. Breast nodules and even the overlying skin often become excessively painful and tender even to light touch until the nodule is proven noncancerous. Children often exaggerate abdominal pain until they are reassured that it is not harmful or serious and will soon go away. Visceral pain is not frequently felt and may be unfamiliar. Familiarity with the pain associated with the surgical incision may cause a deep pain from the area of operation to be referred to the incision. When a pain is familiar, understood, and known or considered harmless, it is more easily tolerated.

Attention and distraction greatly influence perception and reaction to pain. Anticipation of pain seems to make the pain more severe. It is likely that severe shock is analgesic because wounded soldiers often feel little pain before their removal from the battlefield, injured athletes may feel little pain during a contest, and accident victims often feel little pain prior to resuscitation. With less severe degrees of shock distraction probably reduces the perception and reaction to pain significantly.

Memory of a painful experience is poor. Often the subject clearly remembers the unpleasantness of having experienced the painful episode, but the pain itself is poorly remembered. This is a very important point in managing patients with severe abdominal pain. The physician responsible for the therapeutic decisions must examine the patient before narcotics are given because the characteristics of pain are soon forgotten and any associated physical signs may change with pain relief. In life-threatening trauma there is often a short period of unconsciousness followed by a variable period of amnesia.

Pain is disagreeable and to most people unpleasant. (A masochist gets pleasure from pain.) Pain accompanied or followed by *pleasure* is more easily tolerated than pain not associated with pleasure. The pain of childbirth is more easily tolerated than pain caused by unwanted injury.

Fatigue and weariness may distract attention and render pain more tolerable; however, more often self-control and resistance are lowered by fatigue and weariness leading to increased reaction to pain. Rest restores resistance and self-control.

Anxiety, tension, and fear increase the physiological and psychological reactions to pain. Pain tolerance is increased and these reactions are reduced when fear and anxiety are relieved. Often tranquilizers and sedatives greatly reduce analgesic need. As anxiety is relieved, dissociation from pain occurs. Admission to the hospital, the return of mother, and the physician's visit often relieve anxiety and improve pain tolerance. Severe pain is feared while lack of pain causes no fear; this is tragic in the case of the painless breast lump, which is ignored until its persistence, enlargement, and spread signify its seriousness.

Suggestion and reassurance alter reaction to pain. Milder pain may be tolerated better after suggestion by psychotherapy or hypnosis. Strong belief in the successful elimination of pain always makes therapy more effective at least temporarily.

Affect and attitude change during and after painful experience. Persons may become resigned but determined to bear the pain and accept a disability. Alternatively, they may feel angry and vindictive, become fearful, anxious, and irritable or stoic and indifferent to their own and others' suffering. They may become resigned and defeated or more tolerant and kindly toward others. Depression is a common response to chronic pain, and it may reduce or increase tolerance to pain. Intense *religious beliefs* can increase tolerance to pain. *Hysterical* mental states can alter both tolerance and reaction of the subject to pain and color pain description.

Duration of pain alters reaction to it since prolonged pain causes fear, depression, insomnia, anorexia, irritability, and tenseness. Relief of prolonged pain restores emotional balance and improves morale.

Drugs influence pain perception and associated reactions. Analgesics and narcotics raise the threshold for pain. A variety of drugs can alter physiological reactions to pain. Sedatives, tranquilizers, and other mood-changing drugs can alter psychological reactions to pain.

THE PHYSICIAN'S PROBLEMS

In perfect circumstances the physician is able to briefly interview a perceptive, articulate patient and immediately form an accurate concept of the cause of abdominal pain, but neither physician nor patient is perfect.

A physician must acquire *knowledge*. A massive amount of factual and theoretical material is hurled at medical students in their undergraduate years. Often a student is left with the responsibility of deciding what is essential and useful fact and what is theory. Accumulation and consolidation of useful knowledge is the student's primary task.

At the beginning of every physician's career, *experience* is lacking. Despite emphasis early in undergraduate training on having students examine patients, a great variety of problems, both physical and psychological, must be studied before clinical skill is acquired.

Because of work pressures or perhaps because of disinterest in accepting pain as a diagnostic challenge physicians unfortunately tend to be *impatient* and thereby prejudge their patients' problems. Often physicians decide the cause of the complaint too quickly and with insufficient evidence. The physician must listen to the patient's story and extract all possible evidence important in reaching a diagnosis.

In cases of severe pain early diagnosis is essential as treatment is *urgently* required. Because the patient's memory of a pain may be fallacious, analgesics must not be given until the physician responsible for making the treatment choice is satisfied that the patient's history is complete. Answers are needed to a number of questions regarding the characteristics of pain in the abdomen or chest before such pain can be accurately analyzed, and in most instances an accurate analysis is the best way to reach the clinical diagnosis. For example, in the field of gastroenterology 85% of diagnoses are made primarily from the patient's history.

If a physician is essentially *nonsurgical* and has an inadequate understanding of the surgeon's role, the patient may be at greater risk than necessary. There may be delay in treating inflammatory conditions that should be treated as early as possible, such as appendicitis and peritonitis caused by perforation or gangrene. A physician who is persistently (and perhaps subconsciously) averse to surgical care may cause delay in seeking help from consultants most familiar with the care of the severely ill patient, such as patients in shock because of acute pancreatitis, toxic megacolon, or gastrointestinal hemorrhage. Adrenocortical steroids or inappropriate antibiotics may mask the nature of some diseases better treated surgically. There may be tragic delay in the diagnosis of malignant disease, such as gastric, pancreatic, colonic, or bile duct carcinoma thought to be chronic gastric ulcer, chronic pancreatitis, splenic flexure syndrome, or sclerosing cholangitis.

Patients can be subjected to unwarranted risk if their physician has an *excessive surgical orientation*. An operation may be performed because of a wrong diagnosis. Frequently misdiagnosed conditions where the patient is subjected to unwarranted operation include hepatitis, uncomplicated diverticulitis, salpingitis, pancreatitis, and gastroenteritis. Surgical operations may be performed in the absence of disease in cases of malingering, hysteria, Munchausen's syndrome, severe depression, or frank psychosis. Too surgical an attitude can lead to too aggressive treatment for peptic ulcer disease, ovarian cyst, and hiatus hernia to name but a few. The "acute abdomen" or the "surgical abdomen" are unacceptable diagnoses. Any physician should be able to diagnose instances of acute abdominal pain more accurately than these terms indicate. One should be able to recognize at least peritonitis, bowel obstruction, or perforation of a viscus even if the exact cause is unclear. Precise analysis of pain requires knowledge, patience, and impartiality. With greater care in clinical examination and investigation unreasonable diagnoses will be much less frequent. Such uncertain diagnoses for abdominal pain include gastroptosis, cecoptosis, floating kidney, prolapsing gastric mucosa, and sacroiliac subluxation.

Many patients have misconceptions and it is the physician's responsibility to clearly *understand the patient's feelings*. The physician must understand the patient's use of terms such as cramps, colic, tightness, and burning. By listening attentively to the patient's story, the physician has already started treatment since the patient obtains relief from anxiety and fear by telling the story and believing that the physician is paying attention. The physician needs to understand illness and pain. Sympathetic understanding, even in the face of an undiagnosed illness, provides a degree of relief for the patient. The understanding physician should realize that patients wish to please and impress and that they prefer affirmative answers. The accuracy of history taking can be improved by posing some questions that make use of denial. Leading questions should be avoided where possible.

The more *thorough* physician is more accurate than the less thorough. More errors of omission are made than errors of commission. Thoroughness can compensate in part for lack of knowledge and experience.

The uneasiness of not understanding a patient's problem may lead some physicians to make an *impulsive*, early, inappropriate diagnosis. One must resist this tendency and maintain an open mind until enough data are accummulated to justify a reasonable diagnosis.

As new facts are evaluated a physician must be *flexible* and remain willing to change diagnostic impressions or plans of treatment. An inflexible physician persists with an incorrect diagnosis, inappropriate investigation, and fruitless treatment.

Some physicians remain *preoccupied with rare diseases* in an attempt to appear brilliant or search for the unusual to maintain their interest. There is a tendency to become bored with the commonplace. Rarities should be considered only after common diseases have been eliminated. It is more likely for a physician to encounter a common disease with an unusual presentation than a rare disease.

PROBLEMS RELATED TO THE PATIENT

Even if the physician has few difficulties, the problems of understanding the patient and the patient's pain must still be faced. Problems in diagnosis of abdominal pain related to the patient as an individual are discussed below.

Personality Traits

Too often physicians forget that patients are people. Under stress patients tend to show their weaknesses rather than their strengths. Since pain is a sensation, the physician must accept its validity regardless of whether the physician believes it results from organic disease. Patients react to pain between the extremes of pure stoicism and frank hysteria.

The experienced physician learns to evaluate the patient's personality during history taking. When a disorder develops, the personality pattern tends to be similar to the patient's usual personality but some characteristics become exaggerated. Stress causes emotional regression and uncovers underlying weaknesses. A number of personality traits are briefly described below, with the realization that no one person is likely to fall fully into one category. Brief suggestions in managing individuals of each category are given (23, 49).

Long-suffering individuals deny themselves pleasure and suffer to evoke praise. They seem pessimistic, sad, and burdened with the cares of illness. There may be a history of repeated suffering whether from illnesses, disappointments, or other adversities and failures.

With the stress of illness and accompanying emotional regression, complaints worsen, suffering increases, and improvement is denied. As need for love and protection increases, the increasing complaints are maladaptive as they drive most helpers away. Bear in mind that these patients need to suffer. Appeal to these individuals to be as well as possible to reduce the worries of their families and friends.

Attention seekers (hysteric) seek, demand, and exhibit excitable, seductive, and teasing behavior. Because of dramatic or theatrical behavior it is difficult to extract a clear history. With flirtation and sexual suggestions they try to satisfy an insatiable need for affection. In spite of their behavior these immature, insecure, self-centered individuals have a childish wish for nonsexual affection and protection. They are extremely suggestible; care must be taken to avoid leading questions and unwise comments to colleagues that might be overheard.

Hysterics feel that weaknesses are uncovered in their illnesses, and that they are unattractive. Provide professional warmth and friendliness but rigidly avoid emotional entanglement. Listen while these patients satisfy their need to disclose pent-up feelings. Remember that these patients are very sensitive to rejection by others especially authority figures like physicians.

Suspicious (paranoid) individuals suspect the intentions of others. They are stubborn, oversensitive, and tend to be vulnerable, envious, and jealous. They easily feel insulted and isolated and tend to project their weaknesses on others whom they criticize.

When ill they may have a feeling of greater vulnerability, feeling even more inadequate. Avoid argument and maintain a friendly open attitude, explaining their problems and management freely. Take great care to be consistent in answering their questions. Be careful of comments that patients may overhear and misinterpret in a paranoid way.

Self-controlled (obsessive-compulsive) individuals are overly conscientious, concerned with conformity, and set very high standards for themselves. They are diligent, disciplined, show great attention to detail, and tend to be stubborn and rigid in their drives. Ambiguity is intolerable. Defining and categorizing allows everything to be arranged in correct order. Precision, discipline, and attention to detail make them capable of great achievement; however, obsessive-compulsive patients often become depressed.

Obsessive-compulsive patients suffer regression with threatened loss of control of their thoughts and actions. This leads to indecision, fear of poor behavior, isolation, anxiety over their inability to cope, and difficult relationships when these individuals become dependent. Openly discuss the medical problems and management with these patients. Treat the patient as a partner, expecting the patient's help in bringing about recovery.

Individuals with a *superiority complex (narcissistic)* tend to be demanding, arrogant, and self-centered. A sense of inflated importance leads them to believe themselves superior and all-powerful. Such patients willingly compete with anyone including their physicians and look for their physicians' weaknesses in order to exploit them. They are difficult patients to look after, and often make their physicians angry or anxious.

As patients narcissistic people feel their superiority threatened, and their basic feelings of inadequacy come to the surface. Acknowledge the fact that the patient is a person of importance and show respect while directing treatment.

Aloof (schizoid) individuals are quiet, shy dreamers, very seclusive and detached; they try to remain cold and uninvolved and avoid competition and expressions of hostility. Beneath this appearance they are overly sensitive, fearful, fragile, and very easily upset.

Under the stress of illness the schizoid patient withdraws further. Show interest in the individual as a person and give reassurance without retaliation for eccentric behavior. The aloof, remote attitude may create history-taking problems; direct and leading questions may be needed to inquire about specific symptoms.

Antisocial (sociopathic) individuals have superficial relationships tending to aggressive impulses without inhibitions. They have no loyalties but great powers of rationalization. Self-centeredness and callousness do not allow denial of their wished-for pleasures. The pattern of behavior becomes evident in childhood because of lack of discipline, theft, and truancy, always preferring winning to fair play. As adults antisocial persons have poor work records, unstable marital relationships, belligerency, and a tendency to excessive use of drugs and alcohol. The tendency is more frequent in males and tends to decrease in middle age.

When ill sociopaths may become uncooperative and very difficult. They do not trust advice, becoming suspicious, hostile, and antagonistic. Maintain firmness and give positive direction, insisting that the patient carry out orders.

Manic-depressives are characterized by great emotional lability with recurring episodes of elation and depression. In a manic mood they are bright, cheerful, friendly, enthusiastic, energetic, gregarious, and warm. In a depressive mood, they are withdrawn, hopeless, and worried. This leads to pessimism, sadness, and slow behavior.

When ill their lability and variability tend to worsen, but the general direction is toward increasing depression. Be patient and show plenty of encouragement for much is needed by these patients.

The *passive personality* is characterized by dependency, helplessness, and indecisiveness. Such persons avoid responsibility. They try to gain attention to receive affection and to control others covertly.

Emotional regression occurs with illness, and they become more infantile, dependent, and demanding. Supply reassurance and protection but establish limits to the patient's behavior.

Passive-aggressive individuals may appear to perform as requested yet stop before completion with much complaining and passive obstructionism. For example, they may agree to accept treatment but never take it because of complaints or assumptions that it would not work even if it were tried. Supply adequate care. Recognize this as a disorder and avoid punishment. Provide supervision for important treatments.

The *aggressive personality* is characterized by argumentativeness, irritability, and episodes of bad temper. They are overdemanding, believing that they need and deserve limitless care, attention, and advice. If their demands are not met, they become disappointed, angry, anxious, depressed, and frustrated. Their behavior denies or conceals a need for dependency and is maladaptive in that it drives others away preventing the individual from receiving even normal amounts of support, affection, and protection. Be tolerant and supply protection even though it does not appear to be needed. Again, establish limits to the patient's behavior.

An *explosive personality* is characterized by sudden explosive outbursts of aggressiveness by angry verbal or physical behavior. Environmental frustrations excite these patients, and they seem unable to control the outbursts. Try to have their frustrations eliminated as much as possible. Visitors who may upset this type of patient should be restricted.

The *asthenic personality* has low output with little energy, lack of enthusiasm, and difficulty in showing any response to physical or emotional stresses. They seem unable to mobilize resources, feel helpless, and are prone to a wide variety of minor physical complaints especially tiredness. Give more encouragement and support than usual repeatedly pushing your patient toward more normal activity during treatment.

Inadequate personalities seem incapable of any ambition or achievement. Poor judgment, ineptness, poor performance, and poor planning are characteristic. There is a lack of incentive and a tendency to accept menial jobs and handouts. Passive styles of behavior and repeated failure lead to a dull personality. Unemployment, welfare, and failure are accepted as a way of life. Borderline or dull normal intelligence is frequent.

Under stress they appear to be even more helpless. There is not likely to be much of a problem in management although it may be necessary to give more simple directions and explanations than usual.

Simple Neurosis

Simple neurosis, psychoneurosis, or excessive nervousness is often easily recognized. The positive signs of neurosis have been candidly recorded (42). Some patients are sensitive, suggestible, and introspective. Phobias, compulsions, and shyness are common. Adults often give a history of neurosis in childhood and adolescence. There may be a history of nightmares, poor eating and sleeping habits, and difficulty in keeping friends. Broadly speaking, the symptoms affect the whole patient, and common complaints are chronic fatigue, insomnia, morning tiredness, despondency, weeping, and irritability. The psychoneurotic personality is vulnerable to stress. As a rule stress creates fear and anxiety. The normal person responds by sublimation and endurance whereas the psychoneurotic develops an anxiety state, reactive depression, phobias, or obsessional symptoms.

Defense Mechanisms

Defense mechanisms are frequently used by patients to eliminate feelings or thoughts that give rise to unpleasantness. An individual may deny an illness by a statement to the contrary or failure to acknowledge it. Often patients substitute symptoms related to a nearby region when the real problem is feared or considered embarrassing. For example, a woman may complain of shoulder pain when in fact she is worried about a lump in her breast, or a man may have a rectal complaint instead of frankly revealing his sex problem. That which is disagreeable may be suppressed from conscious thought or be repressed so that the patient can neither identify nor accept its presence. Patients may eliminate unpleasant events from their thoughts by rationalization, intellectualization, displacement, or projection. Regression refers to mental withdrawal from unpleasant complexities with a retreat to more simple basic thoughts. Regression may be associated with greater emotional lability and less self-control. As a rule people try to hide their fears. When subjected to stress, fears are uncovered and weaknesses are revealed. Although defense mechanisms were developed to eliminate stress, the fear that the use of these mechanisms might be revealed creates fear and further anxiety.

Anxiety and Depression

In general terms an anxiety state is a reaction to a fear that may be repressed into the subconscious until reappearance is brought about by stress and an association of ideas. Symptoms of the anxiety state then appear in two broad types. The psychological symptoms are an increase in emotional tension and include nervousness, uneasiness, apprehension, irritability, poor concentration, sleeplessness, fatigue, and exhaustion. Psychosomatic reactions are often prominent in anxiety. They include headaches, dizziness, tremors, sweating, palpitations, tachycardia, pallor, precordial pain, shortness of breath, dry mouth, nausea, difficulty in swallowing, vague abdominal pain, diarrhea, urinary frequency, impotence, and skin rashes.

Reactive (exogenous) depression is the response of a psychoneurotic personality to environmental stress and may resemble an anxiety reaction. The early history of the patient's behavior reveals psychoneurotic characteristics with vulnerability to stress. Symptoms often begin with a triggering event and fall into two types. The psychological symptoms include sadness, despondency, self-pity, anger, tiredness, tearfulness, and fatigue with sleeplessness. Severe symptoms such as hopelessness, unworthiness, and self-reproach may precede a suicide attempt. Psychosomatic symptoms include fatigue, poor health, loss of weight, nausea, discomfort or pain after eating, abdominal cramps, and diarrhea. Anxiety and reactive depression can be considered exaggerated but otherwise appropriate responses to changes in the environment.

Endogenous depression arises from within the patient. In the retarded form the individual shows lack of interest in family, friends, and work and becomes withdrawn developing the psychologic symptoms of weariness and fatigue. The psychosomatic symptoms mislead the physician and family since they include constipation, preoccupation with cancer or other serious illness, headache, backache, indigestion, weakness, giddiness, and cramps. Again feelings of guilt, unworthiness, and self-reproach may precede a suicide attempt. In the agitated form of endogenous depression, the individual is overactive and restless. The agitated form of endogenous depression is unexpected, gradual in onset in middle life, and is not caused by any recognized stress from the environment but coincides with illness, convalescence, or menopause.

The more emotionally disturbed the patient, the more difficult it is for him or her to be objective in reporting body sensation. Patients may worry excessively about finances or health. There may be deep anxieties over the preservation of their jobs or deep fears, such as the dread of malignancy, that are often irrational and do not respond to simple reassurance.

Past Experience

The experiences that the patient has had with episodes of pain greatly influence the individual's ability to describe and tolerate a new experience. The athlete may relate a new pain to the pain of trauma, a mother to labor, the laborer to chronic back pain, the elderly to joint pain. The patient may have variations in perception and sensitivity to the same type of pain at different times.

Communications Problem

Some patients are inarticulate. Without coaxing, the patient may hesitate to use similes. Much imagination enters into the patient's description of pain. Very few have felt the pain of a knife stab whereas most have experienced the pain of an electric shock, a tight belt, a heavy weight on the body, or the crampy sensation after taking a strong laxative. Encourage your patient to describe the sensation in any way and then try to decide whether the pain is superficial, somatic, or visceral and whether it is continuous or intermittent. There may be a major language difference between physician and patient. Third persons tend to interpret rather than translate and one can never be sure of the patient's real attitude. As a rule a member of the patient's immediate family is a better translator than an unrelated person. Physicians may also have difficulty communicating with the senile, the aphasic, and the deaf.

Intelligence

The patient may have low intelligence or may be too well informed. A nurse or paramedically trained person has limited medical knowledge and may mislead rather than help the physician. Physicians as patients tend to make early diagnoses and may suggest symptoms to fit them rather than be objective in reporting their sensations. As a patient the physician should behave as a medically untrained individual. When caring for another doctor, assume nothing and provide the same explanation and care as for a non-medical person. Patients of low intelligence should present no greater difficulties than infants and children; recognize their limitations and provide simple explanations.

Need to Impress

Unfortunately many patients feel the need to impress their physicians with the severity of their pain. Some feel that a steady pain should be more severe than intermittent pain; so they report that they feel a continuous pain when they have cramps. Others say that they feel severe cramps when they feel a steady pain, believing that having cramps is more impressive. The most difficult of all are the patients who wish to cover every possibility; they simply suffer both types equally severely.

Secondary Gains

Secondary gains refer to the advantages conferred on the patient by the illness itself. The patient may use pain consciously or subconsciously to influence and manipulate others, gain attention and sympathy, and avoid responsibilities. The gains may include closer attention, financial benefits, and avoidance of unpleasant situations.

The Addict

The narcotic addict may feign illness and plead, fight, beg, or steal for drugs. Experience with doctors and hospitals allows the addict to enact great suffering convincingly. The alcoholic released from inhibitions may delight in mercilessly misleading physicians, nurses, and other attendants. Although specially prone to gastritis, pancreatitis, hepatitis, and chest and head injuries, the alcoholic may be ill from any cause and must be as thoroughly examined as any other patient. Primary care physicians must be familiar with the common symptoms and behavior of addicts and those who abuse street drugs.

PSYCHOGENIC PAIN

Individuals may feel pain that is not caused by recognizable organic disease or injury. Psychogenic pain does not include central pain, causalgia, phantom limb pain, or referred pain. It is believed to arise in the mind. When a breakdown of normal development and behavior occurs, there may be a change in the balanced responses to pain (Figure 2).

As people develop they learn to adapt to life's problems. Intellectual, physical, and emotional development occur more or less together. Individual variations occur because of personality characteristics, parents, relatives, life at home, associations with friends, position in the family, sex of the individual, number of siblings, and many other factors. The normal person wants to have happy relationships with others and behave in such a way as to be rewarded

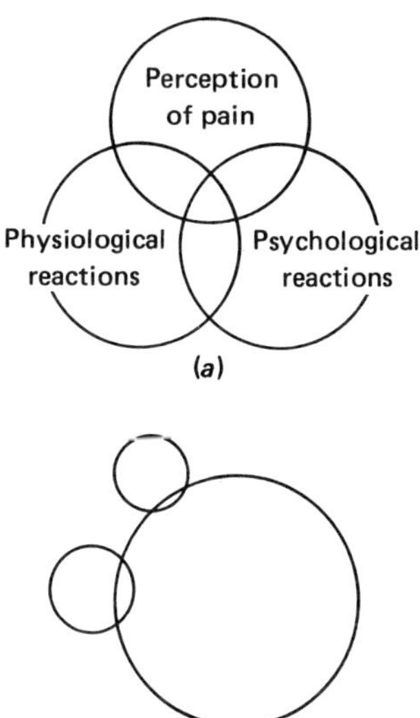

Figure 2 The three attributes of pain (*a*) and the relative changes with psychogenic pain (*b*).

with attention and appreciation. Usually one learns that such attention and appreciation must be deserved.

Unfortunately some individuals do not mature emotionally at the same rate or to the same degree as they mature intellectually and physically. Some individuals cannot accept or resolve their failure to attain their goals in life. Sometimes individuals behave in such a way that they lose attention, appreciation, and love, and some people cannot adapt to these losses. Some cannot adapt to the loneliness caused by the death of a spouse or a parent or the departure of grown children. Others cannot adapt to growing old. These individuals subconsciously convert their lack of adaptation into complaints of poor health. A frequently chosen complaint is pain that is not caused by recognizable organic disease, that is, psychogenic pain. The symptoms and signs that suggest psychogenic pain are as follows:

Inappropriate attitude or behavior
Flamboyant exaggerations
Bizarre symptoms
Inconsistencies
Unrelated multiple symptoms in many systems
Incompatibility with medical fact
Persistence despite potent analgesia or proven block of sensory nerve pathways

Psychogenic pain may fulfill the need to have an acceptable reason for inability to cope with life's problems. Psychogenic pain removes the risk of having inadequacies revealed; it provides a reason for favored treatment or attention so that it is used to manipulate the family. Some individuals want and need the pain. Some physicians believe that there is recognizable gain for the patient who has psychogenic pain. The gain may be the satisfaction of resolving repressed wishes or gaining attention and sympathy and avoiding responsibility (34). Other physicians feel that the importance of secondary gain is negligible and that most patients wish to be released from their suffering (52).

Psychogenic pain problems tend to occur more commonly in widows, the childless, and the unmarried of both sexes. Recurrent psychogenic abdominal pain is frequent in children and adolescents (1). Psychogenic pain is common in the decade following the reproductive years and in early adulthood. Although psychogenic pain is greatest in patients having personality problems and neurotic disorders, particularly hysteria, remember that a neurotic disposition does not prevent one from having organic disease.

The site chosen for psychogenic pain may have a discoverable reason (13). Some patients choose the site where they previously had pain, such as the region of a surgical wound or inflamed organ. Often the patient accepts the site and type of pain suggested by someone else. The patient may have heard of a relative or close friend who has a problem, which the patient readily adopts. Lower abdominal psychogenic pain tends to be related to cramps despite normal bowel sounds and regular bowel habits. Upper abdominal psychogenic pain tends to be associated with anorexia, nausea, and vomiting despite lack of weight loss and dehydration.

The greatest problem is diagnosis. There is no test of high sensitivity and specificity. Patients may have organic disease simultaneously with unrelated psychogenic pain. Nothing is gained by saying that such a pain does not exist. For the individual it does exist and often grows worse as physician after physician attempts to find a diagnosable disease. Although a complete history and physical examination are a necessary part of managing patients with nonorganic pain, stop before ordering a multitude of laboratory investigations. They are expensive, fear-producing for the anxious or depressed patient, and useless because they are likely to produce normal results. It is much better to recognize a nonorganic basis for pain early, but this requires special attention and effort.

Many patients who have psychogenic pain are depressed and have feelings of pessimism and guilt. Some patients are hypochondriacal with many types of pain in many parts of the body. Some are hysterical and the pain is symbolic to the patient. Some are depressed and pain is a symptom of depression or a depressive equivalent. Others are psychotic and delusional.

Recognition and management of psychogenic pain begins with history taking. Be patient and tolerant; otherwise the patient will be defensive. Note especially the dates, times, and circumstances of the onset of symptoms. After carefully noting the patient's story of the development of symptoms, ask more questions to obtain the clearest picture possible. Patients wish to please the interested physician so that affirmative answers are frequent. As stated before, try to formulate answers to make use of denial in order to improve accuracy.

The first suggestion that the patient does not have pain arising from organic disease may be the manner in which the history is given. Patients may be inappropriately relaxed while describing disabling symptoms or may show inappropriate lack of concern. When patients strongly insist that their symptoms must have an organic basis, often they do not. Sometimes patients insist that they are able to tolerate well the symptoms but complain that their families suffer. Symptoms may be described with flamboyant exaggeration. Bizarre symptoms may be described in detail. Inconsistencies may occur on repeated questioning. Unusual developments in the symptoms may be the signal that something is wrong. Organic disease often gives rise to only a few related symptoms whereas patients with psychogenic pain may have a number of unrelated symptoms in a number of organ systems. The fact that the patient has seen a number of physicians beforehand does not necessarily indicate a psychogenic pain, but perhaps a complex organic problem. Nevertheless, if the quality of the previous examinations and investigations is known to be high, it suggests that the patient probably does not have organic disease.

A precise analysis of psychogenic pain on anatomical, physiological, pathological, and clinical grounds is impossible because of incompatibility with medical knowledge. Psychogenic pain might also be anticipated when expected physical and laboratory signs are absent. Failure to admit to any relief with adequate doses of potent analgesics suggests psychogenic pain. Denial of relief of pain with proven block of sensory nerve pathways means that the pain must arise from some level above the block, perhaps in the imagination. Immediate relief when away from spouse, family, home, or work indicates a causal relationship. Similarly relief while in the physician's office or hospital tells much about the nature of the pain.

On careful questioning the precipitating cause can be found in many cases. The individual may be oblivious to the relationship between the psychological stress and the onset of pain. Careful attention to the exact time of onset and association with other events may show that the pain began after a spouse's or parent's death, departure of grown children, illness in the family, financial loss, or promotion of a colleague or junior instead of the patient.

In managing these patients provide understanding and empathy but avoid sympathy and emotional entanglement. A clear explanation to intelligent and receptive patients who are not seriously depressed is often sufficient treatment. If the patient cannot readily appreciate the problem despite explanation, psychotherapy or antidepressant medication may be needed. As a rule analgesics are not helpful alone because some patients need to have pain.

When patients have had previous surgical operations for the same type of pain, be certain there is a clear indication for yet another operation before making that recommendation. One must be certain that symptoms, signs, or other observations have not changed in the interval so that new disease will not be neglected. In their desperation and ignorance of the risks of anesthesia and operations patients may plead for another exploration, believing it to be an acceptable way out of their apparent illness. Psychogenic pain is never a legitimate indication for surgical exploration. When the patient complains of a pain that turns out to be psychogenic, it is not the physician's task to find out why the patient has pain but rather why the patient is complaining.

The accident-prone individual should be distinguished from the pain-prone individual. Accident-prone individuals usually have physical reasons for such behavior, for instance, carelessness, recklessness, incoordination, or sloppiness. Some may be inattentive, irresponsible, demonstrative, easily distracted, or self-destructive. Some may be dull and slow. They may have temporary but often repeated impairment, such as a hangover from alcoholism, or permanent disability in limbs, eyesight, or hearing. Simply by bad luck some laborers experience a series of painful injuries.

MAKING THE DIAGNOSIS

When the history is absolutely characteristic, satisfying all criteria on pain analysis without exception, it is very likely that the diagnosis is correct. Although the patient will be examined and laboratory tests performed, the diagnosis on history alone in this case is sufficiently well established to prescribe treatment. If the history is not diagnostic, characteristic signs on physical examination may be found and these establish a diagnosis. Similarly the history and physical examination may not reveal characteristic features, but a laboratory test may be diagnostic. If the sensitivity of the test is high (high positivity in disease) and its specificity is also high (high negativity in health), the diagnosis is established. Duodenal ulcer may be diagnosed by history alone, inguinal hernia by examination alone, and acute pancreatitis by finding the serum amylase at least five times the upper limit of normal.

In problem cases the evidence from the history, physical examination, and initial laboratory tests is not strong enough to warrant a definite diagnosis; so a series of provisional diagnoses must be considered. These are hypotheses and they are tested by ordering selective laboratory investigations. If the results of such tests are characteristic, then the diagnostic problem is solved. If this evidence like the evidence from history and physical examination is not characteristic, then the available evidence must be reviewed and a working diagnosis chosen. Again this is a hypothesis, and it may be tested by prescribing treatment. Response to treatment is evidence but not proof that the working diagnosis is correct.

The methods by which a physician makes a diagnosis are incompletely understood, having been the subject of study only in recent years. These studies were prompted by the possibility of using statistical analysis with computer assistance in clinical decision making.

Inductive Method

In the inductive method general conclusions are drawn from particular facts. In making a clinical diagnosis the general conclusion is the diagnosis, and the particular facts are evidence from the clinical examination. A thorough clinical examination is completed in every instance by taking a complete history and performing a complete physical examination followed by routine and other appropriate laboratory tests. This method is used primarily for problem cases where facts uncovered from this thorough examination may make possible a diagnosis that might not otherwise have been apparent. This is the method preferred by internists whose lot it is to analyze problem cases. Smith and McWhinney (47) found that internists asked more questions and similar questions more frequently than family physicians, in trial examinations using simulated patients.

Complete history taking and thorough physical examination must be taught sometime, and it is appropriate that the inductive method of making a diagnosis be taught first to undergraduate students of medicine. Shortly, however, teachers should attempt to train their students to constantly evaluate the data as they are revealed and plan investigations earlier and more selectively than the inductive method allows. A comparison of the clinical diagnostic process used by first-year graduates was made with the process used by consultants and postgraduate students in their final years of training (28). These workers found that the first-year graduates used the inductive method. Consultants and senior postgraduate trainees asked fewer questions, asked more significant questions, sought selective physical signs to confirm initial impressions, and reached diagnoses much faster than first-year medical graduates.

The detailed systematic work-up remains the method of choice for the difficult clinical problem. This process protects the physician from the dangers of early hypothesis forming. The danger of early hypothesis forming is inflexibility because it is difficult for a physician to reject a hypothesis once conceived, when there is some confirmatory evidence for it. Evidence supporting a theory may be considered more important than evidence against it. The frequent ambiguity of symptoms and signs may mislead an inexperienced physician to choose hypotheses too early and incorrectly. The stress of responsibility for patient care when the disease is undiagnosed may push many to the security of an early provisional diagnosis before enough clinical facts are appreciated. Adhering to the routine of the classical work-up assures that young physicians not only ask questions to support their favorite hypothesis but also ask questions that afford a thorough and adequate opportunity to disprove it. Furthermore the full routine brings out other facts that could lead to hypotheses other than the initial diagnosis (11).

Teaching clinical diagnosis by the inductive method promotes extensive use of all laboratory facilities. Because there is little critical thinking and professional skill required in regular history taking and physical examination, these tasks might be delegated to specially trained technical assistants. In fact history taking could become a job for the computer (4). At present, medical talent is needed to properly weigh all the facts to reach a provisional diagnosis. Even here, however, it is possible that a properly programmed computer may do the same more accurately and rapidly (39). The inductive method of making a diagnosis remains the mainstay for problem cases, for patients admitted to the hospital where complete medical records are required, and for the initial instruction of medical students learning clinical skills.

The inductive method is less suitable for decision making in investigation. Unselective testing by laboratory methods is wasteful and inefficient. Careful selection of efficient tests of high sensitivity and high specificity must remain the method of choice for laboratory investigation.

Problem-solving Method

In family practitioners' offices, hospital outpatient departments, and the daily care of hospital inpatients, the problem-solving method of diagnosis and therapy is used. In this method the physician forms an early hypothesis before all data are available. From the initial complaints the physician, by a few questions and with a background of knowledge and experience, considers the available clues, identifies the problem, and forms a hypothesis. Such early hypotheses are rank ordered on the basis of (a) probability or frequency, remembering that common things occur most commonly; (b) seriousness, as the most serious problems usually deserve treatment first; (c) treatability, as the most easily treated are more easily dealt with, leaving more time for the others; and (d) novelty, the rare and esoteric are included to maintain interest and to foster exploration of all avenues (11). The physician proceeds to systematic testing along highly selective routes to support these early hypotheses while treatment is given for those problems that require little or no investigation. The testing is designed to identify the disease, its cause, whether it is still operating, the extent and effects of the disease, and the presence of other disease. Another hypothesis or another disease should generate another series of selective investigations (5). Many diagnostic and therapeutic decisions in medicine are based on incomplete data.

Serious disease must be recognized and treated as early as practical. The formulation of hypotheses before all of the data are available, rank ordering of hypotheses, and systematic selective testings are the essentials of the problem-solving method. This is an action method. It promotes solution of complex problems but is partly limited by one's ability to entertain a number of hypotheses simultaneously. Human short-term memory is limited despite almost limitless long-term memory. No more than 7 ± 2 items can be evaluated simultaneously by the human mind (11). Grouping the input by establishing early provisional hypotheses improves data retention.

The problem-solving method uses professional evaluation from the beginning. In this way the interest of the physician is stimulated and in turn the patient appreciates the interest shown. The physician uses a store of acquired knowledge and experience to formulate the hypothesis, calling on an understanding of the frequency, seriousness, and treatability of diseases. It may be decided to examine only certain regions or systems of the body initially, but these are performed in detail to gather as much reliable clinical information as possible. Finally one can be highly selective in using specific tests.

The patient may have symptoms of unrelated disease of secondary importance. This may be missed on incomplete functional inquiry. Many diseases pass through a stage in which they are discoverable on physical examination but have not begun to cause symptoms. These diseases may be missed on incomplete physical examination. Other diseases may have no symptoms, no physical findings, but they may be discovered by simple laboratory tests. Functional inquiry, full clinical examination of the patient, and routine laboratory tests are needed, but these may not play an early role in diagnosis and treatment by the problem-solving method.

Within the problem-solving method there are two subsets. Reasoning may take place in closed or open systems (2).

Goal-seeking Method

In a closed system of reasoning both the starting point and the goal are defined. The aim is to find the most direct and efficient way of reaching the goal. The best choice for appropriate examination, testing, or treatment is based on experience. For example, in the case of a seriously injured patient, the injuries are rapidly defined. The goal is resuscitation and recovery as safely, completely, and quickly as possible. The only problem is to choose the best method of achieving this end.

Highest Yield Method

In an open system of reasoning the end point is poorly defined. The method starts with a hypothesis, the hypothesis is put to the test, and based on the results of the test, with or without newly added data, a new hypothesis is formed. The direction may be straight, but in the absence of a clearly defined ending the method proceeds in the direction that promises the highest degree of success, based on the available evidence. The method requires an open mind because the direction of investigation or treatment may change frequently. An example might be the problem of rapid onset of abdominal pain followed by acute peritonitis. Acute appendicitis was diagnosed first because of the history and the clinical findings. Emergency work-up included plain X-rays of the chest and abdomen, and these revealed free air in the peritoneal cavity. The preoperative diagnosis was changed to perforated duodenal ulcer and the correct incision and operation were performed.

Chance Finding

The discovery of disease by chance is fortunate for the patient. Many diseases are more successfully treated before they have produced symptoms or signs. The chance of such discovery may not be great enough to justify a full work-up on all patients, but this is open to argument. Chance findings are sufficient reason to perform periodic health examinations.

Chance discovery of disease may occur on inquiry into symptoms in systems unrelated to the presenting problem, during physical examination, in multiphasic blood testing, in routine or other laboratory tests, during surgical operation, or at autopsy.

Pattern Recognition

The diagnostic process most difficult to understand is pattern recognition (7). It appears to depend upon recognition of one or more critical discriminatory features. Perhaps the pattern is broken up into parts for analysis, or perhaps the pattern is recognized only as a whole similar to gestaltism in psychology. A spot diagnosis, such as a sucking wound in the chest, a carbuncle on the back of the neck, or a wart on the finger, can be made at a glance. Pigmentation on the lips, melena, and small bowel-filling defects by barium X-ray are typical of Peutz-Jeghers syndrome, a diagnosis made by pattern where there are a cluster of features. Similarly cervical sympathetic motor interruption or Horner's syndrome may be recognized by unilateral ptosis, myosis, anhidrosis, enophthalmos, and flushing. Chapter 8 is devoted to pattern recognition in the diagnosis of abdominal pain.

DECISION MAKING

Diagnosis in the restricted sense refers only to identification of the disease or injury impairing the patient's health. In the broadest sense diagnosis is the identification of disease or injury, the choice of treatment, and an indication of prognosis. These could be called medical decisions rather than diagnoses.

Each decision is based on probability according to the available pieces of evidence or indicants. In clinical diagnosis indicants are derived from the patient's history, the physical examination, or the laboratory tests performed. Clinical decision making is based on the mind's ability to assess weights of evidence or changes in odds based on the available indicants.

Odds and Weight of Evidence

Odds are expressed in numbers, usually fractions, from 0 to infinity. Since the probability of an event is expressed in numbers from 0 to 1, the probability p of no event is $1 - p$. Odds are defined as the probability of an event divided by the probability of no event, p divided by $1 - p$.

A probability of 0.6 means odds are 3 to 2 or the chances are 3 in 5 to 2 in 5. A probability of 1 means that odds are infinite, there is no chance, the result is a certainty. The closer the probability of a disease approaches 1, the greater the odds and the closer the suspected diagnosis approaches a firm diagnosis.

A probability of 0.05 ($p = 0.05$) means that there are odds of 5 to 95 or 1 to 19. This means that the chances are 1 in 20 against 19 in 20. This is a frequently accepted standard that an event is not likely to have happened by chance alone. If the probability were less than 0.05, there would be even less likelihood that the event could have happened by chance alone.

It is fundamental to be able to appreciate the importance of a piece of evidence in diagnosis of a particular disease. The weight of a particular piece of evidence is measured by calculating the change in odds produced by the evidence (39). If the weight of evidence were known for each indicant in every clinical problem, making an accurate diagnosis would be an easy matter.

AIDS TO MAKING A DIAGNOSIS

Probability

Probabilities are derived from making observations of experience over a long period of time to create a reliable data base. This provides a basis for predicting the outcome of actions in a new experience. Published studies have shown the usefulness of probability in the diagnosis of jaundice (26), acute abdominal conditions (6), and dysphagia (9). It has been used in establishing the prognosis of head injury (20), and the success or failure of the medical treatment of acute cholecystitis (48). It has been used in deciding the method of prevention of thromboembolism after myocardial infarction (12), in the treatment of head and neck cancer (17), and in the care of the critically ill patient (46). In each case a few highly discriminative pieces of evidence were used to determine the next best step in diagnosis or management. Only 13 questions were needed to achieve 83% accuracy in the diagnosis of dysphagia (9, 10). In another study (26) 80%, or 52 of 65 patients, could be diagnosed as having medical or surgical jaundice with a probability of 0.96, which corresponds to odds of 24 to 1 that the diagnosis was correct. These accurate diagnoses were made by study of only four criteria: weight loss, abdominal pain, pruritis, and the lack of desire to continue smoking. In a study of acute colitis (48) prediction of success or failure of medical treatment was made on the basis of fever, frequency of bowel movements, serum albumin levels, and pulse rate. It is clear that where the information is available and a correct study is carried out statistical methods can be an aid in making diagnostic and therapeutic decisions for the majority of patients, indicating the small group of patients who require more detailed investigation, and predicting the prognosis when given the needed indicants.

The astute clinician always considers most seriously those pieces of evidence that have the greatest discriminative power and pays little attention to evidence having little discriminative power. Unless there is careful selection, laboratory tests will be performed that have little value and must be considered redundant. It is bad enough to order redundant tests; it is worse to be unaware of the results. If a test is worth ordering, the result is worth the clinician's attention and evaluation.

Decision Trees

Instead of using intuition to make decisions, precedent or previous experience is used to choose the action that appears to have the most to gain and the least to lose. The outcome of the action is one of all possible outcomes. A decision tree can be constructed of nodes that indicate actions and branches that connect nodes and indicate all possible outcomes (45). Decision nodes are controlled as the physician makes the choice whereas chance nodes are uncontrolled. The outcome is shown by one of a number of branches that shows all possible outcomes (28). The decision tree shows options and all possible consequences; it does not indicate the best decision. The best decision is the one with the greatest benefit, greatest safety, lowest cost, or least chance of harm (33). As in games, the treatment is the move by the physician and the outcome of treatment is the move by the patient.

Flow Charts

Flow charts are similar to qualitative decision trees as there is no calculation of probability at each decision node. They are planned to lead from one question or item of evidence to another toward making a diagnosis or ordering investigations or treatment. Such charts are called algorithms. Flow charts and decision trees have been published for guidance in detection and treatment of urinary tract infections (27), treatment of head and neck cancer (17), and diagnosis of dysphagia (9).

Decision Tables

Decision tables were developed by industry as the complexity of manufacturing processes exceeded the ability of management to give directions in simple language. A series of decision charts giving the same information as flow charts on the detection of urinary tract infections has been published (19). Columns and lines show the conditions to be met and the actions to be taken. In these tables an indicator shows what action is to be taken if all of the stipulated conditions are satisfied (41).

Diagnostic trees, flow charts, and decision tables provide a memory aid for the busy practitioner. They can provide a method for history taking by the patient using a prepared sheet or a computer system.

EXPERIENCE AND DECISION MAKING

How can the young physician contend with limited experience successfully? History taking and physical examinations should be very thorough; laboratory testing should be as selective as possible but should always include routine tests for survey purposes. For example, a patient with acute abdominal pain must always have a serum amylase measurement.

It should be remembered that what has worked well in the past will continue to work. Just because something is new does not necessarily mean it is better. Every physician should try to evaluate new proposals critically. Reject former treatment for new treatment only when new treatment has been proven better.

HYPOTHESES, GOOD AND BAD

The benefits of early formation of a hypothesis on incomplete data are evident in the problem-solving method of making a diagnosis. It is to be understood that the next obligatory step is appropriate investigation. Critical analysis of this investigation allows greater confidence in the hypothesis or it may lead to rejection of that hypothesis for another. Adequate testing of the hypothesis and analysis of the test results are essential.

The greatest problem in medical practice is lack of knowledge. Very little is known about the etiology, pathogenesis, and specific treatment of most diseases and unfortunately many physicians forget how little is known. The average clinician has difficulty in separating biological variability and placebo effect from true response to therapy. The natural history of a number of diseases includes remissions and exacerbations. Although there can be no scientific method without the hypothesis, a clear distinction must be drawn between a formulated but untested hypothesis and a tested and accepted one (8, 50). Osler always reminded his students that to distinguish fact from fancy and opinion from stated truth is the most important thing in the practice of medicine.

ACCURACY OF THE DIAGNOSIS

How does a physician know when the diagnosis is right? By pattern recognition the physician may identify an obvious abnormality on clinical examination and as a rule make an accurate diagnosis. Examples include the diagnosis of a fracture by seeing and feeling the ends of the broken bones, prolapsed hemorrhoids, cavernous hemangioma on an infant's forehead, ulcerating carcinoma of the breast, and the rash of herpes zoster. The physician may order or perform one of the few highly specific tests that will establish a firm diagnosis. These include pathological examination of a biopsy specimen, identification of an organism by bacteriological examination, electrocardiographic proof of myocardial infarction, changes in appearance or numbers of the blood cells, and diagnostic appearances on X-ray examination such as an obvious fracture, gallstones, pharyngeal diverticulum, and arterial blockage on arteriography.

The physician may not be able to recognize the abnormality on clinical examination and there may be no diagnostic investigation. If so, evidence should be gathered and a hypothesis formed and tested in various ways. One method is trial of a treatment believed to be appropriate. When improvement is observed, one is led to believe that the diagnosis was correct. But one must not forget that improvement could have taken place by natural healing, use of suggestion, placebo effect, or something the patient has taken or done without the physician's knowledge. Every practicing physician appreciates the value of supportive measures, which include listening to the details of the patient's problem and providing explanation, reassurance, encouragement, and advice. Often the primary care physician examines and treats patients on a single occasion. The physician would expect to hear from the patient if the treatment were unsuccessful, but the patient may have sought the advice of another physician, attended the local hospital, or moved elsewhere. Without an opportunity to analyze the results there can be no evidence to support the hypothesis (14).

Similarly physicians, such as radiologists, who perform and interpret tests for practicing physicians may have difficulty in knowing when they are right. Often they receive little information concerning subsequent investigations or courses of the illness. There are no problems when findings are diagnostic as this implies that the diagnosis is correct. Difficulty arises when the results are suggestive but not diagnostic. These physicians try to help the practicing physician, but they must realize that too much weight may be given to their suggestions by the practicing physician. If the evidence is not strong, the weakness of the evidence should be described. For example, a radiologist might suggest that the gas pattern in the bowel as seen on a plain X-ray of the abdomen of a patient in severe pain looks like paralytic ileus. The practicing physician must remember that the differentiation of paralytic ileus from bowel obstruction rests on clinical evidence and resist being persuaded by the radiologist's attempt to be helpful. The practicing physician must remember that evaluation of the quality of the pain and the exaggeration or suppression of bowel sounds provides firm evidence for the correct diagnosis in this case.

A surgeon is in the privileged position of having immediate confirmation or denial of a diagnosis when internal disease is exposed at operation. This makes the surgeon more perceptive on clinical examination and more critical of clinical and laboratory evidence than nonsurgeons. The exposure of disease at operation, supported by immediate pathological examination, will show whether the preoperative diagnosis was correct. In either case the surgeon has the benefit of comparing evidence for disease with the disease evident.

Medicine is not an exact science. The concept that the practice of medicine and surgery are exact sciences has led patients to expect accurate diagnoses and totally successful treatments every time. It should be clear that much in medical practice rests on probabilities derived from experience with similar problems. Despite the fact that conscientious physicians make every effort to reach accurate diagnoses and prescribe successful treatments, sometimes the diagnosis is not correct and the treatment is inappropriate. Never will the practicing physician harm deliberately, but if the evidence available points to an incorrect diagnosis, it is likely that the treatment that follows will be ineffectual and perhaps harmful. Practicing physicians must remember that it is their duty to explain to their patients any difficulties in making the diagnosis, the probabilities of success of the treatment, and also the possibilities of failure.

In this chapter many of the factors that make the physician-patient interaction difficult have been reviewed. The problems posed by patients as individuals are related to their unique personalities, reactions, and behavior patterns. It is now possible to consider the problem of abdominal pain by more traditional methods. The importance of the patient as an individual does not cease in closing this chapter; the perceptive physician knows that it always remains uppermost in the practice of clinical medicine.

REFERENCES

1. Apley J: The Child with Abdominal Pains, 2d ed. Oxford: Blackwell, 1975.
2. Bartlett FC: Thinking. New York: Basic Books, 1958.

3. Berlin L: Studies of pain; the relation of pain threshold and pain intensity to the phenomenon of extinction. Trans Am Neurol Assoc 229–231, 1953.
4. Card WI: Mathematical method in diagnosis. J R Coll Physicians Lond 9:193–196, 1975.
5. Cox KR: How do you decide what it is and what to do? Med J Aust 2:62–64, 1975.
6. DeDombal FT, Horrocks JC, Walmsley G, Wilson PD: Computer-aided diagnosis and decision making in the acute abdomen. J R Coll Physicians Lond 9:211–218, 1975.
7. Dudley HAF: Pay-off, heuristics, and pattern recognition in the diagnostic process. Lancet 2:723–726, 1968.
8. Dykes MHM: Uncritical thinking in medicine: the confusion between hypothesis and knowledge. JAMA 227:1275–1277, 1974.
9. Edwards DA: Flow charts, diagnostic keys and algorithms in the diagnosis of dysphagia. Scott Med J 15:378–385, 1970.
10. Edwards DA: Discriminative information in the diagnosis of dysphagia. J R Coll Physicians Lond 9:257–263, 1975.
11. Elstein AS, Kagan N, Shulman LS, Jason H, Loupe MJ: Methods and theory in the study of medical enquiry. J Med Educ 47:85–92, 1972.
12. Emerson PA: Decision theory in the prevention of thromboembolism after myocardial infarction. J R Coll Physicians Lond 9:238–251, 1975.
13. Engel GL: Psychogenic pain and the pain prone patient. Am J Med 26:899–918, 1959.
14. Feinstein AR: Clinical Judgement. Baltimore: Williams & Wilkins, 1972.
15. Hardy JD, Wolff, HG, Goodell H: Pain Sensation and Reactions. Baltimore: Williams & Wilkins, 1952.
16. Head H: On disturbances of sensation with especial reference to the pain of visceral disease. Brain 16:1–133, 1893.
17. Henschke UK, Flehinger BJ: Decision theory in cancer therapy. Cancer 20:1819–1826, 1967.
18. Hertz AF: On the sensibility of the alimentary canal in health and disease. Lancet 1:1051–1056, 1119–1124, 1187–1193, 1911.
19. Holland RR: Decision tables. JAMA 233:455–457, 1975.
20. Jennett B: Predicting outcome after head injury. J R Coll Physicians Lond 9:231–237, 1975.
21. Jones CM: Digestive Tract Pain: Diagnosis and Treatment Experimental Observations. New York: MacMillan, 1938.
22. Jones CM: Pain from the digestive tract. In: Pain, Proceedings of the Association for Research in Nervous and Mental Disease, edited by HG Wolff, HS Grasser, and JC Hinsey, pp. 274–288. Baltimore: Williams & Wilkins, 1943.
23. Kahana R, Bibring G: Personality types in medical management. In: Psychiatry and Medical Practice in a General Hospital, edited by N Zinberg, p. 108. New York: International Universities Press, 1964.
24. Kellgren JH: On the distribution of pain arising from deep somatic structures with charts of segmental pain areas. Clin Sci 4:35–46, 1939.

25. Kinsella VJ: The Mechanism of Abdominal Pain. Sidney: Australasian Medical Publ., 1948.
26. Knill-Jones RP: The diagnosis of jaundice by the computation of probabilities. J R Coll Physicians Lond 9:205–210, 1975.
27. Kunin CM: Urinary tract infections. JAMA 233:458–462, 1975.
28. Leaper DJ, Gill PW, Staniland JR, Horrocks JC, DeDombal FT: Clinical diagnostic process. Br Med J 3:569–574, 1973.
29. Lennander KG, Beobachtungen über die Sensibilität in der Bauchhohle. Mitt Grenzgeb Med Chir 10:38–104, 1902.
30. Lennander KG: Über lokale Anästhesie und über Sensibilität in Organ und Gewebe, weitere Beobachtungen II. Mitt Grenzgeb Med Chir 15:465–494, 1906.
31. Lennander KG: Über die Sensibilität der Bauchhohle und über lobale und allgemeine Anästhesie bei Bruch- und Bauchoperationen. Zentralbl Chir 28:209–223, 1901.
32. Lewis T: Pain. New York: MacMillan, 1947.
33. Lusted LB: Decision making studies on patient management. N Eng J Med 284:416–424, 1971.
34. MacBryde CM: Signs and Symptoms, 5th ed. Philadelphia: Lippincott, 1970.
35. Mackenzie J: Some points bearing on the associations of sensory disorders and visceral disease. Brain 16:321–354, 1893.
36. Mackenzie J: Symptoms and Their Interpretation. London: Shaw and Sons, 1909.
37. Melzack R, Wall, PD: Pain mechanisms: a new theory. Science 150:971–979, 1965.
38. Morley J: Abdominal pain as exemplified in acute appendicitis. Br Med J 1:887–890, 1928.
39. Passmore R, Robson JS: A Companion to Medical Studies, vol. 3, chap. 60. Oxford: Blackwell, 1974.
40. Polland WS, Bloomfield AD: Experimental referred pain from the gastrointestinal tract. J Clin Invest 10:435–452, 1931.
41. Pollock SL, Hicks HT, Harrison WJ: Decision Tables: Theory and Practice. New York: Wiley-Interscience, 1971.
42. Rose TF: The positive signs of neurosis. Can Med Assoc J 84:1132–1135, 1961.
43. Ross J: On the segmental distribution of sensory disorders. Brain 10:333–361, 1887.
44. Ruch TC, Patton HD: Physiology and Biophysics, 19th ed. Philadelphia: Saunders, 1965.
45. Schwartz WB, Gorry GA, Kassirer JP, Essig A: Decision analysis and clinical judgement. Am J Med 55:459–472, 1973.
46. Siegel JH, Fichthorn J, Monteferrante J, Moody E, Box N, Nolan C, Ardrey R: Computer-based consultation in "care" of the critically ill patient. Surgery 80:350–364, 1976.
47. Smith DH, McWhinney IR: Comparison of the diagnostic methods of family physicians and internists. J Med Educ 50:264–270, 1975.

48. Spicer CC: The prediction of success or failure of medical treatment for acute colitis. J R Coll Physicians Lond 9:252–256, 1975.
49. Straker M: Comprehensive history taking for the nonpsychiatrist. Can Med Assoc J 96:39–44, 1967.
50. Todd JW: Theory and practice. Lancet 1:33–34, 1972.
51. White JC: Diagnostic novocaine block of the sensory and sympathetic nerves. Am J Surg 9:264–277, 1930.
52. Williams VP: The neuroses in general practice. Med Clin North Am 41:1429–1438, 1957.
53. Wolff AG, Wolf S: Pain, 2d ed. Springfield, Ill.: Thomas, 1958.

FURTHER READING

Bockus HL: Gastroenterology, 3d ed., 4 vol. Philadelphia: Saunders, 1974–1976.

Brooks FP: Gastrointestinal Pathophysiology. London: Oxford, 1974.

Cope Z: The Early Diagnosis of the Acute Abdomen, 14th ed. London: Oxford, 1972.

DeVaul RA, Faillace LA: Persistent pain and illness insistence. Am J Surg 135:828–833, 1978.

Eiseman B, Wotkyns RS: Surgical Decision Making. Philadelphia: Saunders, 1978.

Groves JE: Taking care of the hateful patient. N Eng J Med 298:883–887, 1978.

Guyton AC: The Textbook of Medical Physiology, 4th ed. Philadelphia: Saunders, 1971.

Hannington-Kiff JG: Pain Relief. Phialdelphia: Lippincott, 1974.

MacBryde CM, editor: Signs and Symptoms, 4th ed. Philadelphia: Lippincott, 1964.

Melzack R: The Puzzle of Pain. Harmondsworth, England: Penguin, 1973.

Palmer ED: Functional Gastrointestinal Disease. Baltimore: Williams & Wilkins, 1967.

Sackett DL: Clinical diagnosis and the clinical laboratory. Clin Invest Med 1:37–43, 1978.

Smith LA: Interpretation of abdominal pain, edited by M Paulson, pp. 186–198. Philadelphia: Lea & Febiger, 1969.

Ruch TC, Patton HD: Physiology and Biophysics, 19th ed. Philadelphia: Saunders, 1965.

Way LW: Abdominal pain. In: Gastrointestinal Disease, edited by MH Sleisenger and JS Fordtran. Philadelphia: Saunders, 1973.

Chapter 2

Embryology and Sensory Innervation of the Viscera

Those portions of the central and peripheral nervous systems primarily concerned with the regulation and control of visceral function are collectively termed the autonomic nervous system. As traditionally defined, the autonomic system was a motor system consisting of visceral efferent nerve cells and fibers that passed to tissues other than skeletal muscle. This rigid definition excluded the visceral afferent fibers; yet sensory fibers do in fact accompany most visceral motor fibers and have been shown to form the afferent limb of many visceral reflex arcs. More recently the term "autonomic" has become synonymous with the term "visceral." It should also be noted that visceral innervation is no longer so sharply distinguished from somatic innervation as in the past. Visceral reflexes may be initiated by somatic afferent stimuli and conversely visceral changes may give rise to somatic activities.

The embryonic gut and related structures are derived from endoderm and mesoderm, which are supplied by segmentally arranged autonomic nerves and blood vessels. Both nerves and blood vessels reach the developing gut through the dorsal mesentery. Although this mesentery is not always obvious in the adult because of differential growth and migration of the gut tube, the different parts of the digestive tract and associated viscera retain their original innervation and their original blood supply irrespective of their final adult locations. For this reason logical diagnosis of pain caused by disorders of the gut and its associated glands requires a knowledge of their embryological development including their blood supply and autonomic or visceral innervation, for all are intimately associated from early embryonic life.

Structures that may give rise to abdominal pain include not only the spine and body wall but also the viscera in both the chest and abdomen, together with the pleural, pericardial, and peritoneal linings of these cavities. The viscera that develop in the midline have bilateral innervation; these include the heart, the gut and its related glands, and the spleen.

DEVELOPMENT OF THE HEART

During the third week, the heart begins to develop from mesoderm in the cardiogenic area at the rostral end of the embryo. Paired heart tubes form and fuse into a single midline heart tube. Following flexion of the head end of the embryo, the heart tube comes to lie in a new position ventral to the developing gut in the midcervical area and rostral to the septum transversum. As the heart tube grows it descends into its final position in the thorax, bends to the right, and soon acquires the general external appearance of the adult heart. At the beginning of the fourth week partitioning into chambers begins and is largely complete by the seventh week. About this time autonomic nerves, both sympathetic and parasympathetic, begin to grow into the heart.

DEVELOPMENT OF THE GUT

During the fourth week, the gut is formed from the yolk sac on the ventral aspect of the embryo as a result of longitudinal folding at the head and tail ends and by bilateral infolding in the transverse plane. The primitive gut is derived from both endoderm and mesoderm, the former giving rise to most of the epithelium and glands of the digestive tract while the muscular and fibrous parts are derived from splanchnic mesoderm, which surrounds the endodermal lining.

The epithelium of the primitive mouth, like the lower part of the anus, is derived from surface ectoderm, and both initially develop separately from the gut tube. The primitive mouth cavity, or stomodeum, is separated from the gut by the oropharyngeal membrane, but this breaks down on the twenty-fourth day and so opens the digestive tract to the amniotic cavity. The lower half of the anus is separated from the gut by the posterior portion of the cloacal membrane, known as the anal membrane. This breaks down in the seventh week and establishes continuity of the endodermally derived upper anus with the ectodermally derived lower anus and the amniotic cavity.

Because of this mode of development the ectodermal and endodermal areas at either end of the digestive tract have separate innervation, blood supply, and lymphatic drainage.

That portion of the gut tube that may cause abdominal pain consists of three embryological portions, foregut, midgut, and hindgut. Each has its own discrete segmental blood and nerve supply, which is retained throughout development into adult life, although blood vessels do anastomose and there is some overlap in innervation at junctional areas.

Foregut

The most cephalic part of the gut tube is the foregut, and the cranial portion of this forms the pharynx and the lower respiratory tract and its derivatives. When the embryo is about 26 days old, the primordium of the respiratory tract appears as an endodermal outgrowth from the ventral wall of the foregut. Initially the opening from the foregut into the respiratory diverticulum is large, but this is soon narrowed as the larynx develops around it. The outgrowth forms a midline trachea and then the right and left lung buds. These buds eventually become the main bronchi and divide repeatedly to produce smaller and smaller bronchi and ultimately alveoli. Splanchnic mesoderm around the endodermal outgrowth differentiates into the muscle and cartilage of the respiratory tract, pulmonary blood vessels, and also the visceral pleura around the lungs.

Caudal to the primitive pharynx and the developing respiratory primordium, the foregut first narrows to become the esophagus and then widens to form the stomach and duodenum up to the point of entrance of the common bile duct. A ventral outgrowth of endodermal epithelium into the mesodermal septum transversum gives rise to the liver and biliary apparatus. The pancreas is derived from dorsal and ventral buds of the endodermal cells that arise beside the liver bud from the most caudal part of the foregut. The ventral bud develops into the uncinate process and a portion of the head of the pancreas; the remainder of the pancreas develops from the dorsal anlage. The line of division between the foregut and midgut is marked by the entrance of the common bile duct into the duodenum. Although the spleen is not a derivative of the gut tube, it develops in association with it from mesenchymal cells in the dorsal mesentery of the stomach and likewise obtains its blood supply from the artery of the foregut, the celiac artery.

Midgut

The primitive midgut is open to the yolk sac through the vitellointestinal duct. The midgut begins at the level of the duodenal papilla and extends to the distal transverse colon where it is in continuity with the hindgut. Thus it forms the distal part of the duodenum beyond the ampulla, the jejunum and ileum, the cecum and appendix, the ascending colon, and the proximal portion of the transverse colon.

In the fifth week of development the rapidly enlarging midgut herniates into the extraembryonic coelom within the umbilical cord. During the tenth week, it returns to the abdomen and in so doing undergoes a characteristic counterclockwise rotation of 270° around the superior mesenteric arterial axis. As a result the cecum comes to lie on the right side caudal to the liver and descends to its final position in the right iliac fossa.

Hindgut

The hindgut is continuous with the midgut in the part of the primitive gut that will become the transverse colon. The proximal hindgut forms the remainder of the transverse colon and the whole of the descending and sigmoid portions of the colon.

The caudal portion of the hindgut is dilated and referred to as the cloaca. It extends as far as the cloacal membrane, which separates it from the anal pit or proctodeum. By the sixth week the cloaca is completely divided by the downgrowth of the urorectal septum, which fuses with the cloacal membrane producing separate dorsal and ventral portions of the cloaca. The dorsal portion forms the rectum and the upper half of the anus, while the ventral portion forms the urogenital sinus. The upper half of the anal canal is thus of endodermal origin and derived from the cloaca, therefore sharing its general blood supply and innervation, while the lower half is derived from the ectoderm sharing the blood supply and innervation of the skin around the anal margin.

DEVELOPMENT OF MESENTERIES AND VISCERAL AND PARIETAL MEMBRANES

Certain structures such as the duodenum and the ascending and descending portions of the colon are found on the posterior abdominal wall. All of these structures, like the rest of the bowel, originally possessed a dorsal mesentery, but in the adult it appears that the viscera are firmly attached to the abdominal wall and have lost their mesenteries. The viscera have lain down on the posterior wall and their dorsal mesenteries have fused with the somatic peritoneum that originally covered the ventral aspect of the embryonic dorsal body wall. However, the blood vessels and nerves of the viscus still pass from the midline to the viscus within the original embryonic dorsal mesentery even though it is fused to the body wall and cannot be detected by gross inspection.

The parietal and visceral layers of both peritoneum and pleura are derived separately. While both are mesodermal, the visceral layers are derived from splanchnic mesoderm that coated the gut tube, and parietal layers are formed from somatic mesoderm that lined the inside of the body cavity. It should be appreciated that while the adult ascending colon, for example, is covered with visceral peritoneum of splanchnic origin, on its posterior aspect and lateral border it is in contact with body wall peritoneum of somatic origin. The two layers of peritoneum are adherent and apparently continuous but still possess different nerve supplies that reflect their diverse origins. Visceral peritoneum is supplied by visceral vessels and autonomic afferent nerves whereas parietal peritoneum is somatically innervated and supplied by blood vessels of the body wall. Sensations of pain derived from these two distinct though contiguous layers thus travel by different pathways. They also differ in quality, for pain from somatic layers is bright and sharp while visceral pain is dull, aching, or cramping.

DEVELOPMENT OF DIAPHRAGM

The septum transversum, as its name implies, is a transverse shelf of mesoderm just caudal to the heart. In the fourth week of existence it lies in the midcervical area. It gives rise in part to the central portion of the diaphragm and the liver. The endodermal liver bud, which grows out from the foregut into the ventral mesentery, passes into the septum transversum, and there it rapidly enlarges and divides. The bud thus forms the biliary apparatus and the cords of liver cells while mesoderm of the septum transversum contributes the fibrous, hemopoetic, and Kupffer cells of the liver. After the liver has separated from the remainder of the septum transversum, the latter, together with contributions from the body wall and the dorsal mesentery of the esophagus, forms the diaphragm. As this happens, the diaphragm gradually descends from what will become the neck area to its adult position. In so doing the nerves of the central portion of the diaphragm, which are derived from the third, fourth, and fifth cervical segments descend with it as the phrenic nerves. The peripheral portion of the diaphragm is formed from the body wall and thus is supplied by the same lower seven intercostal nerves that also supply the adjacent body wall.

DEVELOPMENT OF THE UROGENITAL TRACTS

Both the urinary and the genital systems develop from two ridges of intermediate mesoderm that extend along the entire length of the dorsal body wall of the embryo on either side of the dorsal mesentery of the primitive gut tube. Intermediate mesoderm first gives rise to rudimentary pronephric glomeruli in the thorax. Folding and canalization of the epithelial surface of the intermediate mesodermal ridge also gives rise to a series of pronephric tubules that join together to form the pronephric duct that empties into the ventral part of the cloaca (Figure 3).

The pronephric glomeruli and tubules degenerate and, as they do so, are replaced by a second set of glomeruli and tubules, the mesonephros, which lies more caudally in segments T8 to L4. These tubules also open into the pronephric duct. However, with the degeneration of the pronephros and pronephric tubules, the cranial part of the pronephric duct also disappears to the point where the most cranial mesonephric tubule enters it. The remaining caudal portion of the pronephric duct is now referred to as the mesonephric duct. The blind cranial end of the mesonephric duct will become the appendix of the epididymis in the male and the appendix of the epoophoron in the female. The mesonephros is functional in humans during the second and third embryonic months, but it eventually disappears, as did the pronephros, and is replaced by the metanephros.

A ureteric outgrowth arises from the caudal end of the mesonephric duct just before it enters the cloaca. This ureteric bud grows into the intermediate mesoderm, which responds by local proliferation to form the metanephric cap. While the ureteric outgrowth will give rise to the ureter, renal pelvis, major and minor calyces, and collecting tubules, the metanephric cap cells are responsible for the glomerular capsule, convoluted tubules, and loop of Henle. Initially the developing kidneys are found in the pelvis but as a result of embryonic growth in the body wall caudal to the kidneys, they move out of the pelvis. They rise higher and higher in the abdomen and are supplied by arteries and veins at successively higher levels. Usually the caudal vessels degenerate as the kidney ascends and new vessels grow in; however, one or

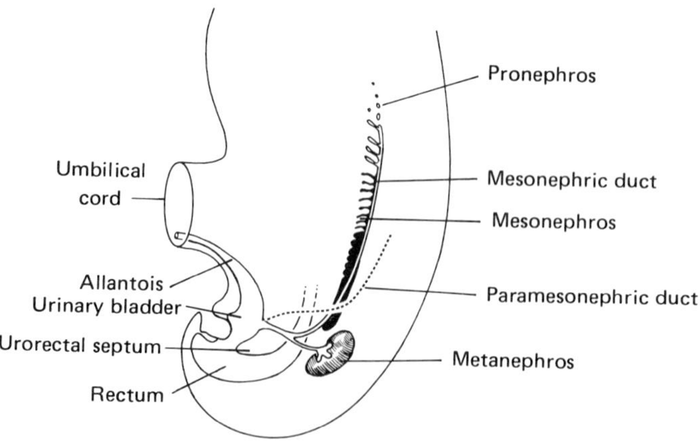

Figure 3 An early stage in the development of the urogenital tract of a 5-week embryo whose crown-to-rump length is 12 mm.

more may persist as accessory renal arteries or veins. After the kidneys have completed their ascent, autonomic nerves grow into them.

During development of the metanephric kidney, the mesonephros degenerates. The cranial mesonephric tubules are taken over by the testis in the male to become the efferent ducts, while in the female they give rise to the epoophoron. Occasionally a few mesonephric tubules remain caudally and these become the paraoophoron of the female. In the male the mesonephric duct loses its renal function, is taken over by the genital system, and gives rise to the epididymis, vas deferens, seminal vesicle, and ejaculatory duct. In the female it remains small and mostly degenerates, but remnants at the cranial, intermediate, and caudal ends may become the duct of the epoophoron, the duct of the paraoophoron, and Gartner's duct, respectively.

Gonads

The gonads develop as proliferations of the epithelium on the medial aspect of the intermediate mesodermal ridge at the level of the first three lumbar vertebrae. Into this proliferation the primordial germ cells migrate from their site of origin in the yolk sac to reach the gonads by the end of the first month. The developing testis descends toward the inguinal canal trailing its blood and nerve supplies behind it, and by the thirty-second week the testis normally enters the scrotum. Similarly the developing ovary descends into the pelvis.

Mesonephric Ducts

When the cloaca is divided into the dorsal rectum and the ventral urogenital sinus, the mesonephric ducts are found to enter the ventral portion. Gradually they are absorbed into the walls of the sinus until even the caudal ends of the ureteric outgrowths have been absorbed. As a result of this process the ureteric orifices are displaced cranially from the mesonephric openings, and the absorbed portions together form the trigone of the bladder. In the male the most caudal part of each mesonephric duct becomes the ejaculatory duct.

Paramesonephric Ducts

The paramesonephric ducts arise in the lateral part of the intermediate mesodermal ridges. Their cranial ends open into the coelom, while their caudal ends cross ventral to the mesonephric ducts to open into the ventral portion of the cloaca between the openings of the mesonephric ducts. Following division of the cloaca, they open into the dorsal wall of the urogenital sinus. Thus the sinus has opening into it the two mesonephric ducts, the ureteric outgrowths, the two paramesonephric ducts, and the midline allantoic diverticulum. The allantoic diverticulum persists as the urachus in both sexes, but the other openings have differing fates.

In the female the caudal parts of the paramesonephric ducts fuse into a common duct, which will later give rise to the uterus and the fibromuscular wall of the upper vagina. The urogenital sinus contributes the endothelial lining of the vagina and its associated glands, the bladder, and the urethra.

In the male the paramesonephric ducts largely degenerate, but small parts remain at either end as the appendix of the testis and the prostatic utricle. The urogenital sinus forms the bladder, the prostate, and the urethra with the exception of the glandular portion.

DEVELOPMENT OF SENSORY NEURONS

At the beginning of the third embryonic week, midline ectoderm overlying the notochord and adjacent mesoderm thickens to form the neural plate. On the eighteenth day, by infolding the neural plate forms the neural folds, which later fuse to form the neural tube, which then sinks below the surface ectoderm. On both sides of the tube are crests containing cells of the neural plate that were not incorporated into the neural tube. Some of these form the sensory or afferent neurons of the dorsal root ganglia and in the cranial region the sensory ganglia of cranial nerves V, VII, VIII, IX, and X (11). Certain other neural crest cells become autonomic ganglion cells and chromaffin cells that form the paraganglia and the medulla of the adrenal gland.

At first the sensory ganglion cells are bipolar, but the proximal portions of the two processes approach each other and thus appear to form a single process that then divides into two. So a pseudounipolar type of ganglion cell is produced whose single process has both peripheral and central branches. The peripheral branches terminate in afferent endings whereas the central branches enter the spinal cord or brain stem depending upon the situation of the cell body. The cell body is invested by satellite cells that are also derived from the neural crest. The embryological development of neuroblasts into dorsal root ganglion cells appears to be identical for both somatic afferent and visceral afferent fibers except for the pathway of their peripheral processes.

PERIPHERAL PATHWAYS OF DORSAL ROOT SENSORY NEURONS

The cell bodies of spinal sensory neurons lie in the dorsal root ganglia. Their peripheral processes pass through the dorsal roots to join the spinal nerves. Those that will supply somatic structures remain within the spinal nerves for distribution by way of posterior and anterior primary rami. The lateral and anterior walls of the abdomen are innervated by thoracic segments 7–12 and the first lumbar spinal nerve; the other lumbar nerves supply the posterior wall of the abdomen. Peripheral processes destined for the viscera have a different route to their destination; they pass by way of the rami communicantes from spinal nerves to sympathetic and parasympathetic ganglia and ultimately form periarterial plexuses. Nerve fibers spiral around the visceral arteries and their branches to reach the viscera (Figure 4).

AFFERENT SYMPATHETIC PATHWAYS

The sympathetic trunks extend from the base of the skull to the coccyx. Some adjacent sympathetic ganglia commonly fuse during development so that the usual number are 3 cervical, 12 thoracic, 4 lumbar, and 4 sacral ganglia, all of which are paired, and the single ganglion impar in front of the coccyx. The sympathetic trunks descend behind the carotid vessels in front of longus capitus and cervicis muscles. In the thorax they cross the necks of the first and second ribs, the heads and radiate ligaments of the lower ribs, and in the lower half of the thoracic region they lie on the bodies of the vertebrae. The trunks enter the abdomen behind the medial arcuate ligaments and descend in the groove between the anterior borders of the psoas major muscles and the vertebral bodies. The trunks enter the pelvis in front of the ala of the sacrum, descend medial to the sacral foramina, and pass medially to join the ganglion impar (Figure 5).

Arising from all of the thoracic and the first two lumbar spinal nerves are white rami communicantes that pass to the sympathetic trunk or its ganglia. They convey the peripheral processes of dorsal root ganglion cells from the spinal nerves to the sympathetic chain. These sensory nerves do not synapse in sympathetic ganglia, however; they pass through them on their way to the viscera that they innervate.

Peripheral processes of sensory nerves may travel up or down the sympathetic chain but eventually they leave the sympathetic chain by way of splanchnic nerves. These nerves also contain other types of autonomic fibers with various functions. From the cervical and the first five or six thoracic segments of the chain, afferent fibers pass to pulmonary, cardiac, esophageal, and preaortic plexuses that lie close to the hilum of the lung, the root of the heart, the wall of the esophagus, and the aorta, respectively.

Although dissection reveals many splanchnic branches from the lower thoracic segments, three large nerves can usually be recognized. Most of the splanchnic branches from the fifth to the ninth thoracic segments of the sympathetic chain join to form the greater splanchnic nerve. Branches from the tenth and eleventh segments form the lesser splanchnic nerve and from the twelfth, the least splanchnic nerve. All run down in front of the vertebral bodies and pierce the crura of the diaphragm to enter the abdomen and reach the preaortic plexus.

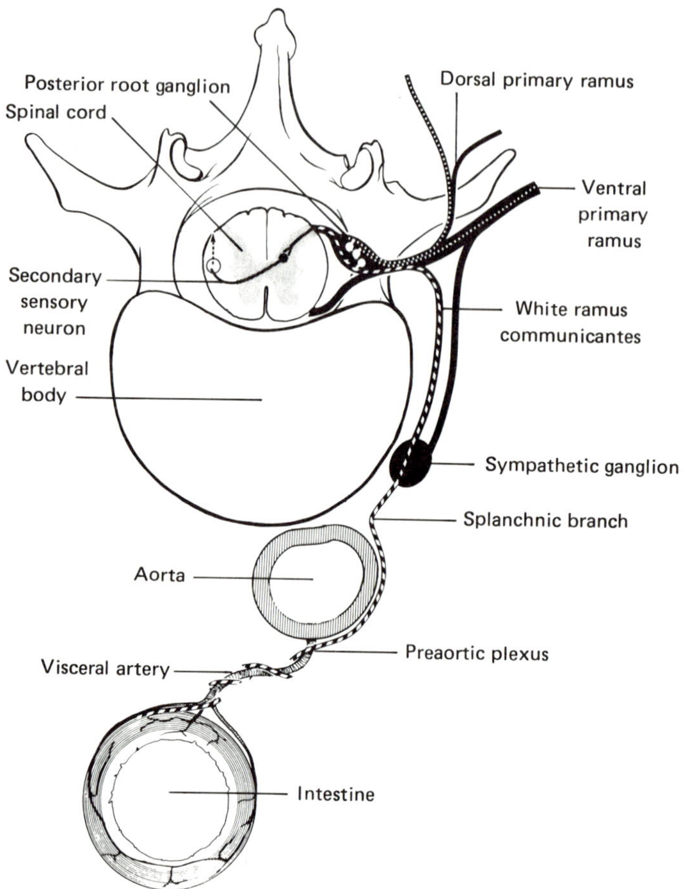

Figure 4 The pathways of the peripheral processes of the cells of a typical posterior root ganglion. Some pass through the spinal nerve to the skin or other somatic structures with the dorsal or ventral primary rami. Others supply the viscera through the white rami communicantes, sympathetic ganglia and trunk, and preaortic plexus to reach a viscus, such as the intentine, by traveling with its artery.

Entering the abdomen then are the sympathetic chains and three named splanchnic nerves on each side together with many small, poorly defined, and unnamed nerves that travel independently or on the esophagus or aorta. With the exception of the sympathetic chain, which continues on into the pelvis, all of the others, including additional branches from the first two lumbar segments, pass to a large, elongated, dense network of nerve fibers and ganglion cells situated on the anterior aspect of the aorta. The network is found not only on the aorta but also on its branches. Although it is not easy to distinguish the different parts of the plexus, it is found to be especially dense around the major

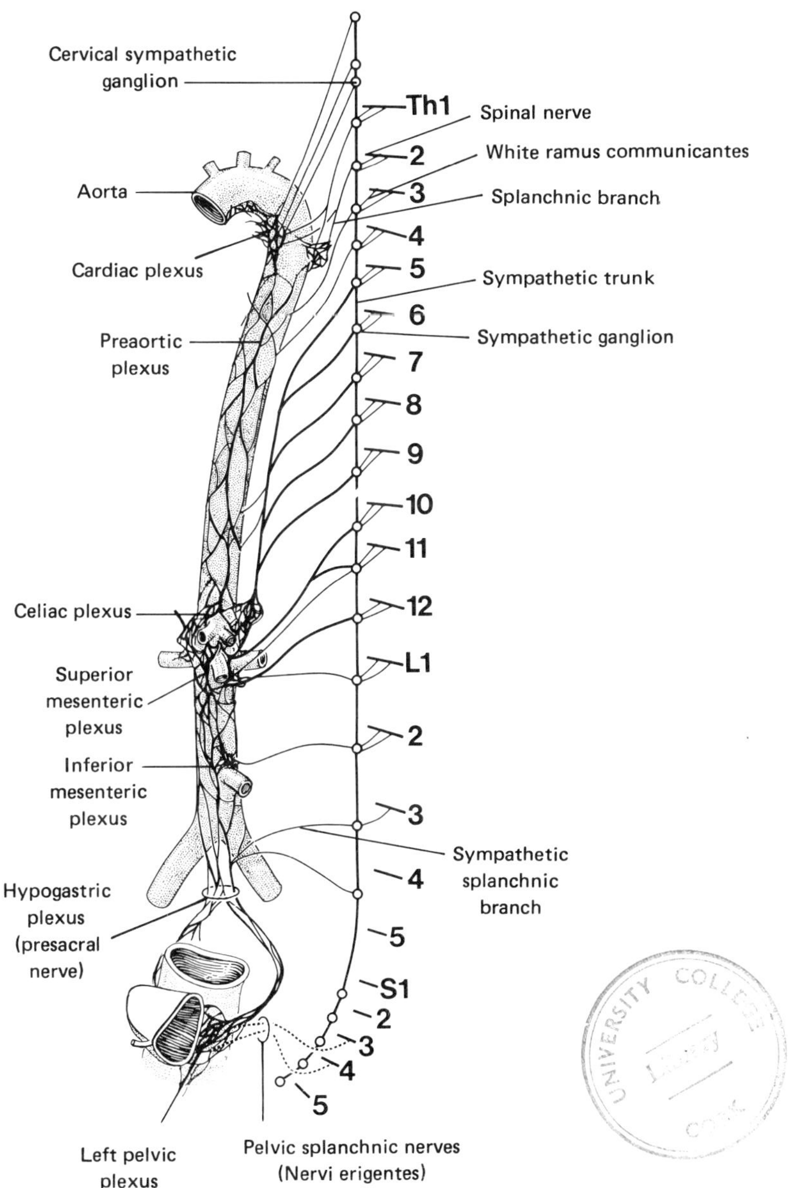

Figure 5 The sympathetic and pelvic parasympathetic nervous systems. Splanchnic branches of the sympathetic system arise from the sympathetic trunk or ganglia whereas the splanchnic branches of the pelvic parasympathetic system arise directly from sacral spinal nerves. Splanchnic branches at all levels are much more numerous than shown. The preaortic plexus is joined also by branches of the vagus nerves.

gastrointestinal arteries; so the plexus is somewhat arbitrarily divided into celiac, superior mesenteric, and inferior mesenteric ganglia.

The abdominal preaortic plexus is continuous with the thoracic preaortic plexus and extends inferiorly to the aortic bifurcation at the level of the fourth lumbar vertebra. The plexus continues inferiorly as the hypogastric plexus, crosses anterior to the aortic bifurcation and sacral promontory, and passes into the pelvis. At the level of the first or second sacral vertebra the hypogastric plexus divides into two, forming the bilateral pelvic plexuses that pass forward on both sides of the rectum and genitourinary viscera (8). Throughout its path the plexus receives additional contributions of both afferent and efferent nerves from the sympathetic trunks.

AFFERENT PARASYMPATHETIC PATHWAYS

The only cranial nerve of relevance to abdominal pain is the vagus nerve. The splanchnic branches of the third, fourth, and possibly fifth sacral nerves must also be included in the parasympathetic afferent system. The cell bodies of primary afferent neurons of the vagus nerve are located in the superior and inferior ganglia, which lie in and just below the jugular foramen, respectively. The peripheral processes of the primary visceral afferent neurons whose cell bodies lie in the superior ganglion pass in the vagus nerve to the dura mater, external auditory canal, and tympanic membrane. All other sensory neurons have their cell bodies in the inferior ganglion. Afferents reach the heart through the cardiac branches of the vagus and the recurrent laryngeal nerves and pass to the cardiac plexus. Other fibers form a large esophageal plexus, and the remaining fibers enter the abdomen as the anterior and posterior gastric nerves. The anterior gastric nerve, derived from the left vagus nerve, sends branches to the stomach, pylorus, duodenum, liver, and pancreas. The posterior gastric nerve from the right vagus nerve sends branches to the stomach and to the celiac plexus for distribution to the structures derived from the foregut and to the superior mesenteric plexus for distribution to the structures derived from the midgut (Figure 6).

The splanchnic branches of the third, fourth, and usually the fifth sacral nerves are called the pelvic splanchnic nerves, or nervi erigentes. They carry afferent fibers, among others, whose peripheral processes pass to the pelvic plexuses and to that part of the preaortic plexus around the inferior mesenteric artery.

ARTERIAL SUPPLY AND INNERVATION OF THE GUT AND RELATED ORGANS

Afferent nerves pass to a viscus as a part of the plexus that spirals around the artery or arteries that supply that viscus. It is important to realize that the

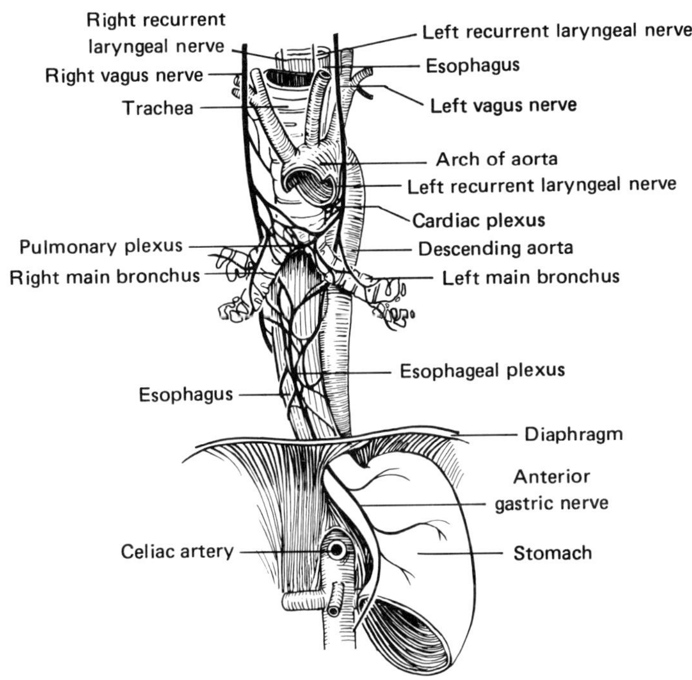

Figure 6 The distribution of the vagus nerve in the thorax. With the exception of the recurrent laryngeal nerves, most of the many branches of the vagus nerves, joined by splanchnic branches of the sympathetic trunk, form the cardiac, pulmonary, and esophageal plexuses. The majority of fibers on the esophagus regroup into the anterior and posterior gastric nerves just above the diaphragm.

embryological segmental level of origin of a viscus largely determines its segmental nerve supply, for nerve processes generally grow into viscera early in their development. Furthermore the nerve supply to each of the various embryological divisions of the gut tube travels with the artery that supplies that section (Figure 7).

The artery of the caudal portion of the foregut is the celiac artery, and nerves from the celiac plexus travel with the artery and all of its branches. All derivatives of the foregut found below the diaphragm with the addition of the spleen are supplied by sensory fibers that pass through the celiac plexus and the vagus nerves. Pain from these viscera appears to be mediated largely by nerves from the fifth to ninth thoracic spinal segments, which travel by the greater splanchnic nerves.

The artery of the midgut is the superior mesenteric artery. Afferent nerves that travel with this artery or its branches to the midgut are derived from the tenth, eleventh, and twelfth thoracic segments through the lesser and least splanchnic nerves with additional contributions from the first lumbar

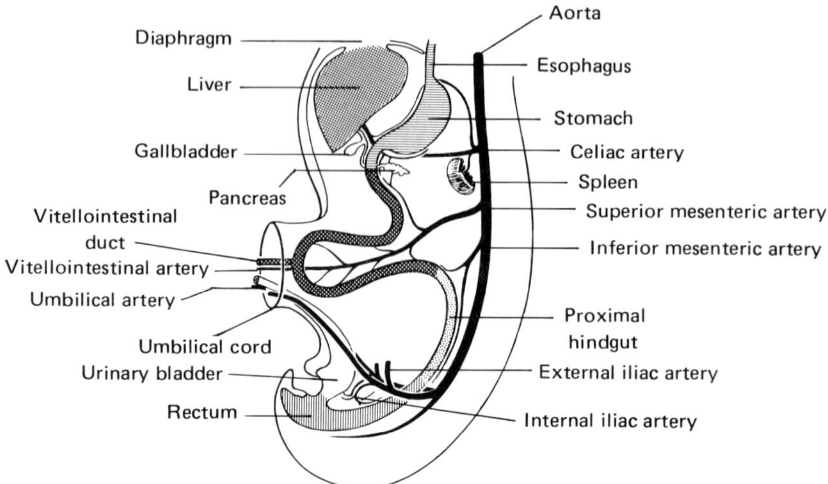

Figure 7 The arterial supply to the embryological divisions of the gastrointestinal tract and related organs. The hindgut is shown divided into proximal hindgut and cloaca, each with its own arterial supply. The embryo is 12 mm from crown to rump at 5 weeks.

splanchnic nerves. There are also fibers from the vagus nerves (5). The pancreas develops at the junction of the foregut and midgut and is thus supplied by branches of both the celiac and superior mesenteric arteries. It is therefore innervated by fibers from both the celiac and superior mesenteric plexuses.

The artery of the proximal hindgut is the inferior mesenteric artery. Nerve fibers to the proximal hindgut arise from the lumbar splanchnic nerves of the sympathetic chain, the superior mesenteric plexus, and branches of the pelvic splanchnic nerves. All of these pass into the plexus around the inferior mesenteric artery and pass with it and its branches to the proximal hindgut. The predominant sensory supply is from the twelfth thoracic and first lumbar spinal segments.

The arterial supply of the distal hindgut and other structures derived from the cloaca is from the paired internal iliac arteries. Nerves that travel in the periarterial plexuses of these arteries and their branches are derived from the hypogastric plexus and the splanchnic branches of the third, fourth, and fifth sacral spinal nerves (8). All of these sources help to form the pelvic plexuses, which pass forward on both sides of the pelvis and spill onto the branches of the internal iliac arteries for distribution. The nerve supply to the distal hindgut and other structures derived from the cloaca is from the eleventh and twelfth thoracic, first and second lumbar, and third and fourth sacral spinal segments. The predominant sensory supply of structures derived from the cloaca is from the third and fourth sacral segments.

GENITOURINARY INNERVATION

Nerve fibers for the kidneys, ureters, vault of the bladder, and gonads can be traced from the tenth, eleventh, and twelfth thoracic, and first and second lumbar segments. Their peripheral processes pass through the spinal nerves, white rami communicantes, sympathetic trunk, and splanchnic nerves, including the least splanchnic nerve, to reach the preaortic plexus and the renal plexus surrounding the renal artery. From here they travel along the renal or gonadal arteries to their destination. The sensory supply of the kidney and ureter is from the tenth thoracic to the first lumbar segments. The sensory supply of the testis and ovary is mainly the tenth and eleventh thoracic segments.

The base of the bladder, prostate, cervix, and upper vagina, like the rectum and upper anal canal, are derived from the cloaca and are supplied by the internal iliac arteries. Nerves supplying these structures can be traced through the hypogastric and pelvic plexuses from the splanchnic branches of the sympathetic trunks and the third, fourth, and possibly the fifth sacral nerves. The vault of the bladder is supplied through the hypogastric plexus with sensory fibers derived from the eleventh and twelfth thoracic segments and the upper two lumbar segments. The body of the uterus is supplied through the hypogastric plexus and mainly by the twelfth thoracic and first lumbar nerves.

SEGMENTAL INNERVATION OF VISCERA

The distribution of spinal nerves to the skin of the body is shown in Figure 8. Although not obvious in the adult the viscera are similarly innervated by afferent nerves from various spinal nerve levels so that they too have a segmental supply. This segmental distribution has a very important bearing on the location and distribution of pain arising from the viscera. The segmental distribution of cranial and spinal nerves explains how pain may be referred to apparently remote areas of the body, areas that are supplied by other branches of the same spinal nerve. Spread may occur to adjacent segments usually in a cranial direction.

The segmental innervation of the viscera has been studied by a variety of methods. Human anatomical dissection (10, 15, 18) has its limitations since microdissections are difficult and time consuming and there is variation in fine detail. Nerve blocks in humans have confirmed most pathways (13, 21). Similarly operations under local or regional anesthesia provide the observant surgeon with accurate information (1, 9, 12, 13, 16). Experiences with unilateral and bilateral resections of portions of the sympathetic trunks or splanchnic nerves for control of idiopathic hypertension or intractable pain have been reported (20, 22). Patients with various gastroenteric stomata (2,

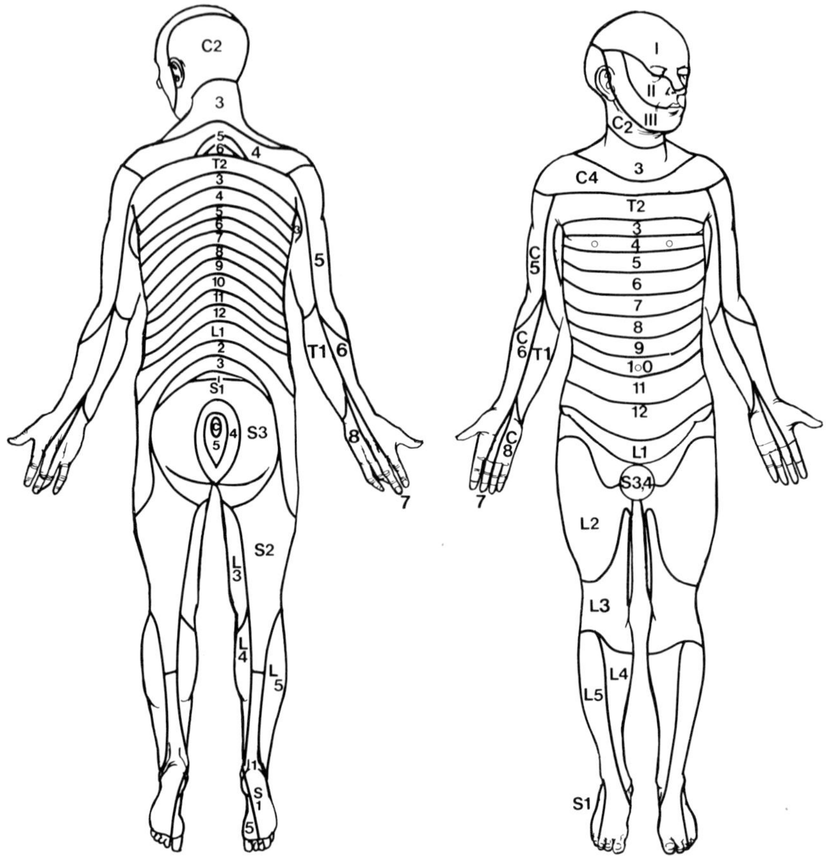

Figure 8 The sensory distribution of the three divisions of the trigeminal or fifth cranial nerve and spinal segments to the skin.

23) and human volunteers who have reported their sensations after distension of balloon tubes (6, 7, 19) have been studied in detail. Slight variations in the segmental innervation of viscera have been reported by different authorities, but this should be expected because of the variety of sources and because of prefixation, postfixation, and multiple interconnections (1).

The predominant sensory segmental innervation of the abdominal viscera described above is based on our experience and careful study of the available literature. However, rather than concentrate on the segmental levels that appear to supply various viscera, the student is urged to study the patterns of innervation through periarterial plexuses, the usual distribution of pain, and the areas of pain referral from the various viscera; they will be most helpful in understanding a patient's complaint of abdominal pain (Tables 1-3).

Table 1 Segmental Innervation of Skin, Walls of Body Cavities, and Viscera

Segment		Surface area	Parietes	Viscera
Cervical	2	Back of head		
	3			
	4	Top of shoulder	Central diaphragm (C3–5)	
	5	Outer arm		
	6	Thumb, outer forearm		
	7			
	8	Fifth finger		
Thoracic	1	Inner forearm		
	2	Inner arm		Heart, esophagus (T1–6)
	3			
	4	Nipple		
	5		Thoracic walls (T1–12)	
	6	Xiphoid		Thoracic aorta (T3–12)
	7			Derivatives of foregut (T5–9)
	8	Epigastrium	Anterior and lateral ab-	
	9		dominal walls (T5–L1)	
	10	Umbilicus		Testis, ovary (T10, 11)
	11			Derivatives of midgut (T10–L1)
	12	Hypogastrium		Kidney, ureter (T10–L1)
Lumbar	1	Groin		Vault of bladder (T11–L2)
	2		Posterior abdominal wall	Derivatives of proximal hindgut (T12, L1)
	3	Front of knee	(L1–4)	Body of uterus (T12, L1)
	4			Abdominal aorta (L1–4)
	5	Great toe		
Sacral	1	Fifth toe		
	2	Posterior thigh		
	3		Pelvic walls (S1–5)	Derivatives of cloaca (S3, 4)
	4	Midsacrum		
	5			
Coccyx	1	Tip of coccyx		

Table 2 Sensory Innervation of the Viscera

	Viscera	Artery	Nerve plexus	Primary pain	Referred pain
Heart	Heart	Coronaries	Cardiac	Central chest	Shoulder, arm, neck
Esophagus	Esophagus	From aorta	Esophageal	Central chest	Midline back
Foregut	Stomach, pancreas, liver, gallbladder, proximal duodenum	Celiac	Celiac	Midepigastrium	—
Midgut	Distal duodenum, jejunum, ileum, ascending and transverse colon	Superior mesenteric	Superior mesenteric	Umbilicus	—
Proximal hindgut	Descending and sigmoid colon	Inferior mesenteric	Inferior mesenteric	Hypogastrium	—
Gonads	Testis, ovary	Gonadal	Renal	Gonad	Umbilicus
Proximal urinary	Kidney, ureter	Renal	Renal	Costomuscular, loin	Groin, scrotum, labia
Bladder, body of uterus	Bladder, body of uterus	Internal iliacs	Hypogastric	Hypogastrium	Groins
Cloaca	Rectum, upper anus cervix, upper vagina, base of bladder, prostate	Internal iliacs	Pelvic	Midpelvis	Midsacrum

Table 3 Segmental Innervation of the Walls of the Body Cavities and Predominant Sensory Innervation of the Viscera

	Cervical							Thoracic												Lumbar					Sacral				
	2	3	4	5	6	7	8	1	2	3	4	5	6	7	8	9	10	11	12	1	2	3	4	5	1	2	3	4	5
Parietes																													
Central diaphragm		3 ←		→ 5																									
Thoracic walls								1 ←											→ 12										
Anterior and lateral abdominal walls												5 ←								→ 1									
Posterior abdominal wall																				1 ←			→ 4						
Pelvic walls																									1 ←				→ 5
Viscera																													
Heart								1 ←					→ 6																
Esophagus								1 ←					→ 6																
Thoracic aorta										3 ←									→ 12										
Derivatives of foregut												5 ←				→ 9													
Testis, ovary																	10–11												
Derivatives of midgut																	10 ←			→ 1									
Kidney, ureter																	10 ←			→ 1									
Vault of bladder																		11 ←			→ 2								
Derivatives of proximal hindgut																			12 ←	→ 1									
Body of uterus																			12 ←	→ 1									
Abdominal aorta																				1 ←			→ 4						
Derivatives of cloaca																											3–4		

CENTRAL CONNECTIONS FOR PAIN

After entering the cord the central processes of dorsal root ganglion cells branch into short ascending and descending fibers. They synapse in the dorsal horn of the gray matter with secondary sensory neurons. These are common to both somatic and visceral pain, and may be an explanation for referred pain (17). Almost all central fibers of the second neuron cross the midline to the opposite side of the cord within a few segments and ascend in the lateral spinothalamic tract. The remaining pain fibers ascend in the multisynaptic pathways in the dorsal columns, in the lateral spinothalamic tract on the same side, and in the dorsolateral tracts (14, 17). Central connections are probably in the brain stem reticular formation for the most part, and other fibers pass to the hypothalamus, limbic system, thalamus, and cortex. Little is known about the central connections of the vagal afferents.

ANATOMICAL BASIS FOR ABDOMINAL PAIN

The gastrointestinal viscera originally develop in the midline and have bilateral innervation so that in the adult visceral pain is interpreted as coming from the midline rather than from the position of the viscus (3). Thus pain from the gut tube or its derivatives is felt in the epigastrium if it arises from the foregut, umbilical region from the midgut, hypogastrium from the proximal hindgut, and pelvis from structures derived from the cloaca. Spinal nerves that send pain fibers to the viscera have other branches carrying sensory fibers, and the pattern of distribution of these branches gives an anatomical explanation for the phenomena of referred pain, muscle guarding, hyperalgesia, and hyperesthesia (Figure 9).

Pelvic structures are innervated by lumbar and sacral segments below those segments supplying the anterior and lateral abdominal walls so that one should not expect to find muscle guarding, hyperesthesia, or hyperalgesia in the abdominal wall when disease is confined to the pelvis.

Cardiac pain is felt deep in the center of the chest, but it may be felt throughout the distribution of the branches of the cervical sympathetic ganglia in the neck and face. Pain is also felt in the skin areas supplied by the first and second thoracic segments on the medial aspect of the arm and forearm and especially on the left side.

Pain from chest disease may be felt as if it arose from the abdomen because of the obliquity of the thoracic segments. Similarly pain resulting from disease in the upper abdomen may be felt as if it arose from the chest; for example, visceral pain from gallbladder disease is felt in the midline of the epigastrium as biliary colic and may be referred to the interscapular region in the back. Somatic pain of acute cholecystitis is felt in the right upper guadrant of the abdomen and may be referred to the inferior angle of the right scapula.

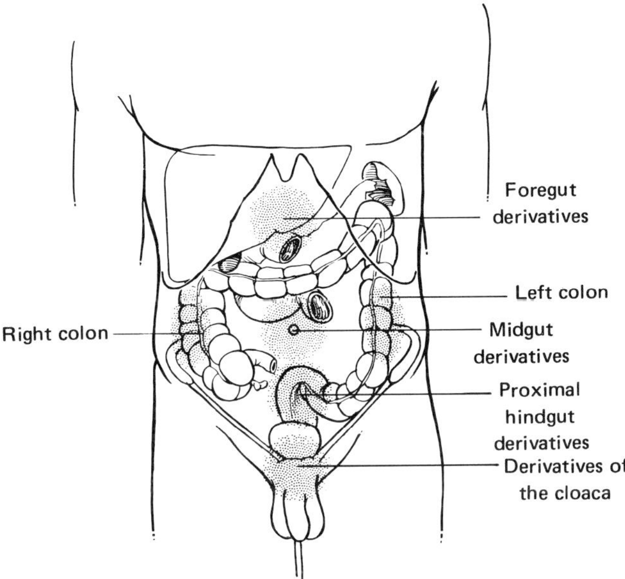

Figure 9 Visceral pain from most parts of the gastrointestinal tract is felt in the midline at four levels that are related to the four embryological divisions of the tract. The exception is visceral pain from the right or left side of the colon that may be felt in the right or left flank, respectively.

Pain arising from deep structures in the body including the walls of the body cavities is generally well localized and lateralized. The kidneys and ureters have unilateral visceral innervation so that pain is felt on the same side as the injury or disease causing the pain (4).

Knowledge of the embryological development of the viscera and their nerve and arterial supplies is most helpful in understanding the distribution of abdominal pain. Patterns of abdominal and referred pain and associated phenomena can only be understood on this basis.

REFERENCES

1. Adson AW: Splanchnic pain. Mayo Clin Proc 10:623–624, 1935.
2. Beaumont W: Experiments and Observations on the Gastric Juice and the Physiology of Digestion, 1833. Facsimile of the original edition. Boston: XIII International Physiological Congress, 1929.
3. Brown FR: The problem of abdominal pain. Br Med J 1:543–546, 1942.
4. Brown FR: Testicular pain. Lancet 1:994–999, 1949.
5. Charney KJ, Juler GL, Comarr AE: General surgery problems in patients with spinal cord injuries. Arch Surg 110:1083–1088, 1975.

6. Hertz AF: On the sensibility of the alimentary canal in health and disease. Lancet 1:1051–1056, 1119–1124, 1187–1193, 1911.
7. Jones CM: Digestive Tract Pain: Diagnosis and Treatment. New York: MacMillan, 1938.
8. Kimmel DL, McCrea LE: The development of the pelvic plexuses, and the distribution of the pelvic splanchnic nerves in the human embryo and fetus. J Comp Neurol 110:271–297, 1958.
9. Kinsella VJ: The Mechanism of Abdominal Pain. Sidney: Australasian Medical Publ., 1948.
10. Kuntz A: The Autonomic Nervous System, 4th ed. Philadelphia: Lea & Febiger, 1953.
11. Langman J: Medical Embryology, 3d ed. Baltimore: Williams & Wilkins, 1975.
12. Leriche R: Des douleurs provoquées par l'excitation du bout central des grands splanchniques au cours des splanchnicotomies. Pr Med 45:971–972, 1937.
13. MacIntosh R, Bryce-Smith R: Local Analgesia: Abdominal Surgery. Edinburgh: Livingstone, 1962.
14. Melzack R: The Puzzle of Pain. Harmondsworth, England: Penguin, 1973.
15. Mitchell GAG: Anatomy of the Autonomic Nervous System Edinburgh: Livingstone, 1953.
16. Morley J: Abdominal pain as exemplified in acute appendicitis. Br Med J 1:887–890, 1928.
17. Passmore R, Robson JS: A Companion to Medical Studies. Oxford: Blackwell, 1974.
18. Pick J: The Autonomic Nervous System. Philadelphia: Lippincott, 1970.
19. Polland WS, Bloomfield AD: Experimental referred pain from the gastrointestinal tract. J Clin Invest 10:435–452, 1931.
20. Ray BS, Neill CL: Abdominal visceral sensation in man. Ann Surg 126:709–724, 1947.
21. White JC: Diagnostic novocaine block of the sensory and sympathetic nerves. Am J Surg 9:264–277, 1930.
22. White JC, Sweet WH: Pain and Neurosurgeon. Springfield, Ill.: Thomas, 1969.
23. Wolf S, Wolff HG: Human Gastric Function—An Experimental Study of a Man and His Stomach. London: Oxford, 1943.

FURTHER READING

Adriani J: Labat's Regional Anaesthesia, 3d ed. Philadelphia: Saunders, 1967.

Hollinshead WH: Anatomy for Surgeons, 2d ed. New York: Harper & Row, 1971.

Hannington-Kiff JG: Pain Relief. Philadelphia: Lippincott, 1974.

Johnson RH, Spaulding JMK: Disorders of the Autonomic Nervous System. Oxford: Blackwell, 1974.

Langman J: Medical Embryology, 3d ed. Baltimore: Williams & Wilkins, 1975.

Mitchell GAG: Anatomy of the Autonomic Nervous System. Edinburgh: Livingstone, 1953.

Moore KL: The Developing Human, Clinically Oriented Embryology, 2d ed. Philadelphia: Saunders, 1977.

Morley J: Abdominal Pain. Edinburgh: Livingstone, 1931.

White JC, Smithwick RH, Simeone FA: The Autonomic Nervous System. New York: MacMillan, 1952.

White JC, Sweet WH: Pain and the Neurosurgeon. Springfield, Ill.: Thomas, 1969.

Chapter 3

Physiology of Abdominal Pain

Many years ago it was appreciated through observations made on skin stimulation that there were two primary types of pain: bright, sharp, well-localized pain and dull, vague, poorly localized pain. Various authors identified these types of pain as epicritic and protopathic, fast and slow, phylogenetically new and old, and heavily myelinated and poorly myelinated (13). Bigelow, Harrison, Goodell, and Wolff (3) believed the difference was a result of two different qualities sensed by characteristic receptors, whereas Lewis (12) and Gasser and Erlanger (7) believed the difference occurred because the two sensations were carried in different fibers at different speeds. More recently sharp pain has been explained as being carried rapidly by generously myelinated large A-delta fibers (1–4 micrometers in diameter) conducting impulses at a speed of 5–15 meters per second and dull pain as being carried by unmyelinated or sparsely myelinated smaller C fibers (0.5–1 micrometer in diameter) conducting impulses at a speed of 0.5–2 meters per second (8). The majority of pain fibers are C fibers rather than A fibers. Another explanation for the two types of pain is that the sharp early pain results from mechanical stimulation and the slower more prolonged pain results from chemical stimulation of the same receptors.

If one pinches, then squeezes, the sensitive skin fold between the base of the fingers or flips the back of the finger near the nail bed against a hot light bulb, one can appreciate a sudden, bright, early pain sensation followed by a more vague, prolonged, slower aching sensation. The threshold for these two types of pain becomes dissociated in certain conditions. Mild hypoxia causes an elevation of threshold for fast pain but a lowering of threshold for slow pain. Similar threshold changes occur in most types of peripheral neuritis and in nerve injuries such as pressure on nerve roots by an extruded intervertebral disc. Local anesthetic agents affect the relatively unprotected C fibers before the myelinated, well-protected A fibers.

Action potentials are the electrically measurable changes in nerve fibers as an impulse is transmitted. It is generally believed that the action potentials in peripheral nerve fibers always have the same amplitude; therefore, if different sensations are transmitted in the same nerve, they must be discerned by variations in frequency.

PAIN FROM DEEP STRUCTURES

As described in the historical note in the first chapter, it was shortly before the beginning of this century that surgeons began careful observations on the types of pain that arose from deep structures in the body. It became clear that pain arising from viscera had qualities similar to the slowly propagated, dull, protopathic type of pain that can arise from stimulation of the skin. To further complicate the terminology, it was realized that nonvisceral deep pain, for example, pain arising from ligaments, tendons, and joint capsules, could be dull and aching similar to visceral pain, or it could be quite sharp and clearly localized similar to the sharp pain arising from stimulation of the skin.

Considering the quality of pain alone, there are only two primary types: bright, sharp, epicritic pain and dull, vague, protopathic pain. However, considering the apparent origins of pain, there are four categories: superficial pain (essentially epicritic), visceral pain (essentially protopathic), deep pain, and central pain (both deep and central pain are mixtures of epicritic and protopathic).

Superficial pain arises from stimulation of the surface of the body by stimuli from the environment. This pain is clear, bright, sharp, acutely perceived, well localized, usually familiar, and generally easily explained. It is an alerting sensation and is appreciated as the main sensation resulting from injury.

Visceral pain is the only type of pain, in fact the only sensation, that arises from internal viscera. It is dull, poorly localized, usually unfamiliar, and generally unexplainable by the patient. It tends to cause inactivity and is appreciated as a threat to health by noxious stimulation within the body. Visceral pain is also called splanchnic pain.

Deep pain originates in nonvisceral deep structures in the body and is caused by disease or injury. The quality of this pain is a mixture of the qualities of superficial pain and visceral pain in that it may be sharp and well localized, or dull and poorly localized. Deep pain may arise from joint capsules, ligaments, tendons, muscles, nerves, blood vessels, or the linings of body cavities. In general it is better localized, lateralized, and more clearly described by patients than visceral pain; unfortunately a more definitive term has not been generally accepted. Deep pain arising from musculoskeletal structures, nerves, and blood vessels is often called somatic pain, and that from the walls of body cavities is often called parietal pain.

Central pain occurs where there is no peripheral representation or where the peripheral representation is lost or damaged. Disease of the cerebral cortex or major nerve tracts may cause central pain. Causalgia results from damaged peripheral nerve trunks. Most instances of central pain result from pain persisting after a peripheral stimulus has ceased: phantom limb pain persists after the amputation of a limb; the pain of herpes zoster may persist long after the rash has cleared and even after peripheral nerve blockade by infiltration of local anesthetic agents.

QUALITY OF PAIN

Pain as described by the patient varies with many factors including the patient's past experience, emotional control, objectivity, language facility, and imagination. There are a few characteristic terms such as gnawing for peptic ulcer, tearing for dissecting aneurysm, boring for bone pain, compressing or constricting for angina pectoris and myocardial infarction, lightninglike or shooting for tabes dorsalis, and pounding for aneurysmal erosion of bone. More often than using these terms, the patient chooses terms from his or her imagination colored by attitude and emotional state.

Lewis (12) was among the first to subclassify superficial and visceral pain. Bright, sharp, superficial pain may be instantaneous, best described as a prick. In fact there is a sudden, bright, sharp prick followed by a dull after-pain of lesser intensity. The second type of bright superficial pain is continuous and has a constant intensity generally described as a burning sensation. Another superficial pain is a variant of a burning sensation where there is regularly fluctuating intensity coinciding with the pulse; this is described as a throbbing sensation.

Visceral pain is dull and vague; continuous visceral pain is often described as a steady aching sensation. The other type of visceral pain is a colic that has a varying intensity, rises to a peak, persists for a short period, then subsides and disappears completely until the next colic begins. The cycle tends to recur at $1\frac{1}{2}$–4-minute intervals in intestinal colic. Colic can be very severe; patients who have experienced severe intestinal colic would never describe their pain as dull or aching in character.

TIME-INTENSITY CURVES

Lewis (12) described the time-intensity curve to graphically illustrate the qualities of pain. This concept can be an aid to appreciating which basic type of pain the patient feels. Further evidence for diagnosis comes from pain analysis rather than from more detailed description of the qualities of the pain by the patient. The diagrams indicate the manner in which the pain starts, the rapidity of its culmination, the duration and smoothness of its height, and the manner of its decline (Figure 10).

Most patients can give their physicians some indication of the severity or intensity of the pain by relating it to some painful experience in the past. When properly questioned, patients can indicate the duration of the pain and whether it is steady or intermittent. Most patients are able to decide whether the pain is superficial or deep, once their physician points out the qualities of these two types of pain.

With regard to cramps, colic, or the constancy of pain the physician should be certain of understanding what the patient actually feels rather than accepting the patient's descriptive terms without question. Often the patient choses whichever type of pain seems most impressive.

PAIN-SENSITIVE STRUCTURES

The mucosa of the gastrointestinal tract consists of glandular epithelium from the lower end of the esophagus to the middle of the anal canal. Glandular

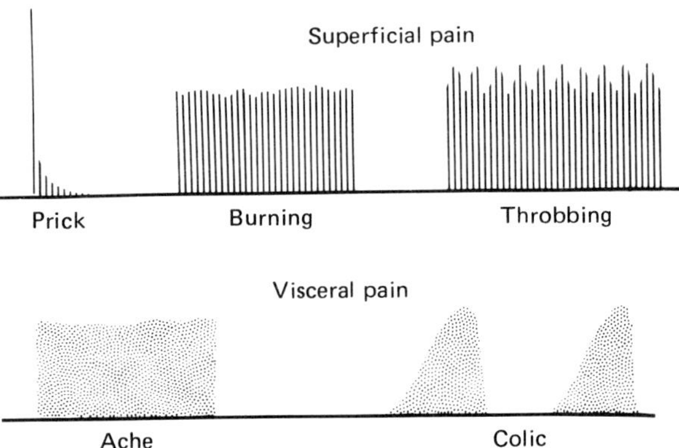

Figure 10 Time-intensity curves for superficial and visceral pain. Nonvisceral deep pain consists of a mixture of most of the qualities of superficial and visceral pain.

epithelium is insensitive; squamous epithelium above and below these limits is sensitive to most of the stimuli to which the skin is sensitive. The walls of hollow viscera, visceral peritoneum, and the adjacent mesentery are insensitive to most stimuli except an increase in tension by stretch, sustained muscle contraction, or ischemia. The root of the mesentery and the parietal peritoneum are sensitive to most mechanical, chemical, thermal, and electrical stimulants.

In order to make a differential diagnosis of abdominal pain it is important to understand pain arising from other parts of the body. The dorsal nerve root is a pain sensitive structure, as demonstrated by the pain caused by pressure from a herniated intervertebral disc, osteoarthritic osteophyte, or extramedullary tumor. Spinal nerves may give rise to pain because of neuritis, neoplasm, or fracture of a rib. The skin is very sensitive to all painful stimuli. In the subcutaneous tissues the only pain-sensitive structures are the sensory nerves and blood vessels. The intima and media of larger vessels are insensitive but the adventitia is highly sensitive. The adventitia is covered by the periarterial plexus of sympathetic efferent and afferent fibers as well as visceral sensory fibers for pain; this is the route whereby pain fibers reach the viscera. The capsules of solid viscera cause pain when they are stretched, and therefore rapid enlargement or distension of solid viscera causes pain whereas slow enlargement is painless. Tendons, ligaments, fascia, and periosteum are sensitive to needling, squeezing, and increased tension by swelling or stretching. Muscles become painful because of sustained contraction, swelling, or the accumulation of metabolites as a result of decreased blood circulation and anoxia. Synovial membrane is sensitive but articular cartilage is insensitive.

PAIN PERCEPTION THEORIES

There are three main theories of pain perception. The specificity theory postulates that pain is the result of activation of a special subsection of the nervous system in which pain involves specific receptors, peripheral fibers, and central tracts. In such a system a specific stimulus should elicit a predictable reproducible response. The second theory is the pattern theory, which assumes that specific nerve end structures for pain do not exist but that the sensation results from the activation of general receptors in a special pattern for pain. The pattern is decoded by the cerebral cortex and pain is appreciated. The third theory postulates a gate or valve mechanism in the posterior horns of the spinal cord capable of modulating the stimulus (10). Thus the stimulus may be augmented or inhibited before central transmission occurs. Discussions of other theories may be found in the references and further readings for this chapter.

PAIN RECEPTORS

The end organ for the reception of stimuli that cause the sensation of pain is the free nerve ending of the branching dendrites of primary afferent neurons.

Bare nerve endings are also known to give rise to the sensations of pressure and temperature change. However, some nerve endings are receptors for pain alone, as they are found in some viscera sensitive to pain but insensitive to pressure and temperature change.

Bare nerve endings occur in densities that vary among the pain-sensitive organs. Nerve endings are very dense with much overlapping of fibers in skin and squamous epithelial mucosa at the body orifices, less dense in parietal peritoneum, the root of the mesentery, and parietal pleura. Pain receptors are sparse in the visceral peritoneum of the hollow viscera and in the adjacent mesentery and in the capsules of solid viscera. There is very little overlapping of pain fibers in these structures. No nerve endings for pain are found in either the parenchyma of the central nervous system or the lungs; both appear to be insensitive to pain.

PAIN STIMULUS

A number of stimuli—chemical, mechanical, electrical, extreme heat or cold—can give rise to the sensation of pain. Not all pain receptors react to pain alone; many receptors react to other stimuli and produce a pain response only with intense stimulation. For instance, mechanical or chemical stimulation causes the sensation of pain whenever the intensity approaches the point where the stimulus might produce tissue damage. Thus the threshold for pain is close to the threshold for tissue damage. If the stimulus continues, tissue damage results. Pain indicates continuing tissue damage rather than amount of damage. Once tissue is dead, it is insensitive.

Injury to tissue causes release or formation of several pain-producing substances, such as plasma globulin, various polypeptides, histamine, and serotonin or 5-hydroxytryptamine. In high concentration these substrates cause pain directly; in lower concentration the pain threshold is lowered, a characteristic feature of inflammation. Armstrong, Jepson, Keele, and Stewart (1) demonstrated that inflammatory exudates and blister fluid can form a globulin and a polypeptide resembling bradykinin or kallidin, which are pain-producing substances. Chapman and others (5) identified a polypeptide termed neurokinin obtained from sites of migraine headache. They also found a protease that they felt was responsible for the formation of neurokinin from plasma precursor substances. Blood serum appears to produce pain when injected extravascularly because of the serotonin it contains. Nettle stings contain pain-producing concentrations of acetylcholine, histamine, and serotonin. Wasp venom has a high concentration of histamine, serotonin, and various polypeptides, which are perhaps the chemical agents responsible for pain. These may constitute the pain-producing metabolite referred to by Lewis (9).

The abruptness of the onset of pain caused by injury is in keeping with a physical or electrical rather than a chemical reaction. The injury probably changes membrane permeability, creating an electrical potential and an electrical impulse that travels rapidly.

Stimulus for Visceral Pain

Visceral pain is produced by increased tension in the wall of a hollow viscus, ischemia, or rapid enlargement of a solid viscus. Balloon distension of a hollow viscus in an unanesthetized human volunteer causes pain (9, 14). These observations are easily repeated by balloon tubes passed by mouth or rectum into colostomies, ileostomies, cholecystostomies, and other stomata or fistulas. Rapid distension of a hollow viscus causes pain and a strong contraction of the muscle wall. Slow distension is pain free and the reflex muscle contraction in response is weak.

Smooth muscle has the properties of self-excitation, spread of excitation from cell to cell independent of innervation or secretion of an excitory substance, rhythmic contraction, and tonic contraction. The strength–duration curve of smooth muscle resembles that of skeletal muscle but the chronaxie is longer. Under physiological conditions local or remote neural stimulation is the main stimulus for smooth muscle contraction. The only reflex arc in the body that can act independent of the spinal cord or brain occurs in the autonomic innervation of the gut. Smooth muscle contraction may be stimulated by local mechanical factors of which stretch appears to be the most important (8). Stretching and pinching are easily demonstrated stimuli during laparotomy, endoscopy, and radiological examination.

Visceral pain caused by smooth muscle stretch or contraction is considered to result from muscle ischemia or accumulation of acid metabolites, drugs, or hormones. Smooth muscle contraction is stimulated by cooling or by an increase in concentration of hydrogen ions, lead salts, histamine, acetylcholine, pilocarpine, and vasopressin. Strong stimulation by these agents causes either crampy or steady pain. Ischemia causes steady pain in smooth muscle similar to ischemic pain in skeletal muscle. Pain appears earlier if the muscle is in use at the time of stimulation. Muscle pain with ischemia and hypoxia is associated with sustained muscle contraction and local accumulation of acid metabolites; it persists until circulation is restored or the muscle dies.

Although stretch is the main mechanical stimulus for smooth muscle contraction, the response is modified by innervation, hormones, and chemicals. In many parts of the body smooth muscle has a double nerve supply, sympathetic and parasympathetic. Responses are often antagonistic and depend upon the release of two different substances, acetylcholine and norepinephrine, and the type of response varies in different parts of the body. Some smooth muscle has sympathetic nerve supply only, for example, the walls of arteries and veins in the limbs. Smooth muscle of the uterus is greatly influenced by hormones.

Peristalsis and Paralytic Ileus

When the intestine is exposed at laparotomy, continuous irregular contractions are seen. This inherent rhythmic contractile activity, paralytic ileus, continues in the postoperative period; it is not effective peristalsis. Once contractions become coordinated, active propulsive peristaltic activity resumes and bowel sounds can be heard as swallowed air is churned with liquid bowel contents. The reappearance of bowel sounds, passage of gas by rectum, reduction of the volume of fluid aspirated from the stomach, and lessening of abdominal distension signal relief from paralytic ileus. Coordinated regulation of smooth muscle activity by the return of nervous control is the reason for the return of normal peristalsis and may be encouraged by sympathetic inhibition and mild parasympathetic stimulation by suitable drugs (4).

PAIN THRESHOLD

The threshold for pain is the minimal stimulus for the perception of pain. It may be raised or lowered by a variety of psychological factors or by analgesics and epinephrine. Pain threshold is lowered by local tissue damage, inflammation, hyperemia, anoxia, and ischemia. The threshold for pain is at or close to the threshold for tissue damage, which is believed to be approximately the same for everyone in good health (16) although reactivity to pain varies greatly.

LOCALIZATION OF PAIN

The ability of a subject to appreciate the source of pain varies with the density of nerve endings in the irritated tissues. Localization depends also on the subject's familiarity with the pain; for example, the ulcer patient or the arthritic patient can identify and locate the familiar distress with ease. When a new pain arises from an unfamiliar site, it may be associated with a referred pain usually felt on the surface of the body and always in tissues supplied by branches of the spinal nerve innervating the site of the original pain. Localization is always related to the distribution of the spinal nerve; difficulties arise because as a rule part rather than the entire distribution of the spinal nerve is involved. There is a tendency for deep pain, when it is severe, to give rise to projection of pain to a superficial area, a referred pain. The reverse can take place; for example, injection of concentrated sodium chloride solution into an interspinous ligament can cause visceral pain within the same spinal segment; injection of the C8–T1 interspinous ligament produces pain indistinguishable from angina pectoris (15).

There may be difficulty in accurately localizing the site of a painful condition. The patient's history may be faulty because of misunderstanding or difficulties in communication; the memory of a pain is faulty once the pain has disappeared. Summation may cause pain to be felt in an area not identifiable with the most important cause. An early postoperative pain may be referred to a clean incision or to another area because of a lingering deep infection. Many of the spinal segments have wide and varied distribution. The foregut is innervated by the fifth to ninth thoracic spinal nerves but these spinal nerves also innervate part of the chest, esophagus, and heart. The midgut is innervated by segments T10-L1, but these segments also supply the chest and abdominal walls. The proximal hindgut is innervated by segments T12-L2 and these segments also send afferent fibers to the kidneys and ureters. Whenever spread to adjacent spinal segments occurs it tends to occur in a cranial direction.

LATERALIZATION

Parietal pain is well localized and lateralized; it remains on the same side of the body with few exceptions. One of the exceptions is left upper quadrant abdominal pain felt by about 1 patient in 24 who have early cholecystitis without pancreatitis.

An embryological midline viscus such as the gastrointestinal tract has bilateral innervation so that visceral pain from the various gastrointestinal viscera is felt in the midline. As a general rule pain arising from an intraperitoneal viscus is felt in the midline, whereas pain from retroperitoneal or parietal tissues is better localized and lateralized to its own side of the body. Dworken, Biel, and Machella (6) showed that distension of the splenic flexure of the colon could give rise to pain in the left costal margin, precordium, border of the left trapezius muscle, and inner side of the left arm resembling angina pectoris. This pain was immediately relieved by decompression of the bowel by an enema. It is believed that this visceral pain is felt on the left because of stimulation of parietal peritoneum on the left side of the abdomen.

SEVERITY

The severity of pain involves not only the intensity of the pure sensory phenomenon but also the physiological and psychological reactions to it. In general the psychological reactions to pain are less reliable indicators of severity than the physiological reactions, with involuntary more reliable than voluntary reactions. Inflammation causes almost all body tissues to become more sensitive to pain and more sensitive to less intense stimulation (16).

Try to appreciate the severity of the pain by a general appraisal of the patient–nature, complaints and attitudes, facial expression, pallor, frowning, clenched jaws, body position, body movement, dryness of mouth, change in blood pressure, change in pulse, perspiration, or change in temperature of the skin. Examples of how the body position or body movement might indicate the severity of pain are the immobile supine patient with peritonitis, the curled-up, writhing patient with colic, the immobile patient protective of a part with a painful musculoskeletal disorder, and a sitting patient supporting the epigastrium with the forearms or bent-up knees because of pain in the region of the pancreas. Involuntary muscle contraction, such as splinting of abdominal wall muscles, indicates a more severe pain than voluntary muscle contraction of the anterior abdominal wall muscles.

CHARACTERISTICS OF THE SYNAPSE

Most of our information on nerve transmission has come from studies of the reflex arc. The arc includes the receptor of the stimulus, the transmission of the stimulus in the afferent neuron, the synapse, the efferent neuron, and the effector of the response. It is assumed that most of the characteristics of the afferent–efferent synapse are the same as the characteristics of the primary afferent–secondary afferent neuron synapse because many of the characteristics of one can be applied to the other on the basis of clinical observations.

Adaptation

A weak stimulus may not produce a response. As the intensity of the stimulus increases, the frequency of action potentials increases so that the receptor is capable of a variable response to a greater range of intensities. If the stimulation is constant and prolonged, the response decreases and adaptation occurs. If the stimulation is slowly increased, adaptation to it may prevent noticing the increase. The rate of change of the stimulus must be faster than adaptation in order to stimulate the neuron to transmit the impulse.

Convergence and Divergence

The terminal fibrils of a number of primary neurons may synapse with one secondary neuron, called convergence, or one primary neuron may synapse with more than one secondary neuron, called divergence. There is a measurable but very short delay at the synapse, which appears to be capable of one-way transmission only.

Facilitation

Facilitation, the mechanisms of which are poorly understood, suggests that either the resistance at synapses is lowered or the central threshold for pain perception is reduced in frequently used pathways. Facilitation is influenced by past experience, learning, and habit. In the Jones experiment (9), if there was a surgical scar, balloon distension in the intestine always produced a visceral pain, not in the midline, but in the operative scar. Similarly abdominal pain may persist for a time after its cause has been corrected; for example, a deep right upper quadrant abdominal pain may persist for a period after successful cholecystectomy.

Summation

Two stimuli received close together may have an additive effect. If two terminal fibrils each carry a stimulus, neither of which would result in a propagated sensory impulse, and these synapse with the same secondary neuron, an impulse might be propagated because of spatial summation. Similarly if two subliminal impulses arrive at the synapse through the same terminal fibril in sequence, the second closely following the first, an impulse may be propagated and temporal summation is said to have occurred.

Summation may explain some unusual relationships. Part of the pain of angina pectoris may be somewhat relieved by antacids in patients who also have mild reflux esophagitis (10). The pain of duodenal ulcer disease is occasionally partially and temporarily relieved with emptying of the colon. Heartburn, gastric distension by air swallowing, and colonic distension by gas can produce a great variety of widespread discomforts in susceptible individuals. It is probable that there are a number of terminal fibrils that are incapable of activating a secondary neuron; however, a pathway becomes established through which one fibril takes advantage of the effect of the arrival of another fibril's impulse. Facilitation takes place because of spatial summation. Facilitation may explain the hypersensitivity of central nervous system centers after repeated stimulation. Perhaps repeated cortical stimulation contributes to the hypersensitivity of patients with chronic rheumatic pain who become sensitive to atmospheric temperature, pressure, and humidity changes.

Intensity

The intensity of pain is related to several circumstances. Although increasing the area of painful stimulation may not greatly increase the intensity of the pain, the overall effect is one of a more widespread and therefore more serious pain. If two pains are present, the pain intensity is no greater than the more intense pain. Because the peripheral processes of afferent neurons branch, a single neuron innervates a larger area than would be possible if it had but one nerve ending. There are few neurons in viscera in contrast to the large numbers in the skin, and there are fewer nerve endings in the visceral peritoneum than in the parietal peritoneum. There are many more primary neurons than secondary neurons (11), which may help to explain referred pain (15). The additive effect of a number of subliminal stimuli produces pain when the pain threshold is passed.

Inhibition

Inhibition, the opposite of facilitation, describes the apparent capability of some presynaptic neurons to raise the threshold of excitation, thereby reducing the chance that impulses carried by other neurons will pass through the synapse. This physiological observation may explain the clinical observation of extinction where one pain can raise the threshold for perception of a subsequent pain. Extinction may explain the success of counterirritants, pain control by electrical counterstimulation, and the effectiveness of acupuncture (2).

CENTRAL EXCITORY STATE

The central excitation produced by converging stimuli from a number of primary afferent neurons in a region has led to the concept of a central excitory state. There is a prolonged, sustained irritation capable of causing other phenomena, such as facilitation, lowering of the pain threshold, and hyperalgesia within the affected spinal segments. Wolff and Wolf (16) found that infiltration of a local anesthetic agent into an area of hyperalgesia could modify the severity of the pain but that the pain would not disappear until the site of stimulation was anesthetized by another injection. An area of hyperalgesia may be located in skin, muscle, tendon, or ligaments; anesthetizing these trigger points with a local anesthetic agent usually relieves much of the original pain.

In a similar way the central excitory state may be responsible for stimulating the contraction of skeletal muscles, which, if sustained, may cause pain by itself. When the innervation of these muscles is blocked by local anesthestic agents, the muscles relax and this pain is relieved. However the original pain causing the central excitory state remains unless the original site is anesthetized.

THREE ATTRIBUTES OF PAIN

The three types of responses of the body can be applied to superficial, visceral, and somatic pain (Figure 11).

Superficial Pain

Superficial pain may be instantaneous or continuous and, if continuous, the intensity may be constant or fluctuating. It gives rise to the sensations

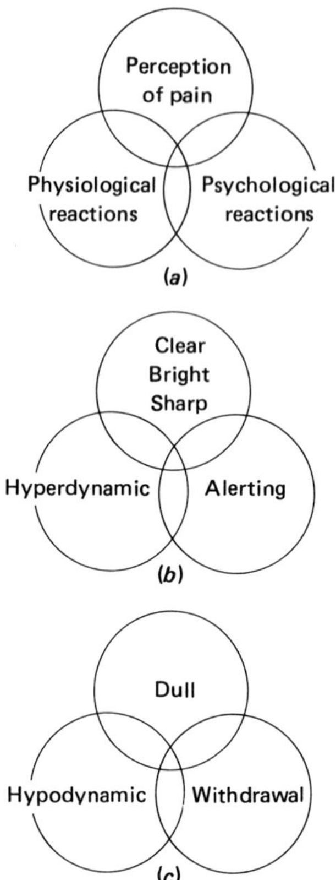

Figure 11 The three attributes of pain (*a*) as they relate to superficial (*b*) and visceral (*c*) pain.

commonly called a prick, a burning, or a throbbing. Superficial pain is caused by a stimulus from the environment, a pain from without. The reactions to such a pain alert the person to prepare for flight or fight.

The physiological reactions to superficial pain are both autonomic and physical. The autonomic response resembles sympathetic motor stimulation in that the heart beats faster and blood vessels undergo constriction in many areas to increase peripheral resistance and raise the blood pressure. Blood is shunted from the skin and intestines to the heart and skeletal muscles; the pupils dilate. The respiratory rate may increase; yet the depth decreases in keeping with the general tensing of skeletal muscles. Withdrawal by releasing a noxious object is a physical reaction. There is a tendency to flex joints and tense skeletal muscles in preparation for activity. It is interesting that the withdrawal reflex, a primitive spinal reflex, remains intact in the decerebrate experimental animal. There is release of epinephrine, and in general a stimulation of defense mechanisms.

The psychological reactions to pain vary with the circumstances and the surroundings. The person becomes more alert and aware, part of the preparation to face or flee the threat. Fear, apprehension, or a sense of danger are common responses.

Visceral Pain

Visceral pain may be continuous or intermittent and is felt as an aching dull pain or a colic. Visceral pain may be described by patients as sharp in the sense that it is severe but not superficial. Visceral pain is generally unfamiliar, unexpected, and poorly localized. The term colic is often used by patients interchangeably with the term intestinal cramps. However, the term cramps also refers to tonic spasm of skeletal muscles, such as calf muscle cramps. It is important to clarify the patient's intention when these terms are used.

The physiological reactions to visceral pain are both autonomic, resembling a vasovagal response, and physical. The heart rate slows and the blood pressure drops. There is vasodilation and decreased peripheral resistance. Salivation is frequent and nausea and vomiting may occur. The patient perspires, feels generally weak, and is usually immobile except in instances of colic when the patient tends to roll about and groan. It should be appreciated that the physiological reactions may lead to a failure of defense mechanisms.

The psychological reactions to visceral pain vary with the patient's understanding of the problem. Visceral pain suggests a threat from within the body so that the patient becomes concerned with self and develops self-pity. The patient becomes inattentive to the surroundings, becomes dependent, perhaps shows resignation or withdrawal. The feelings caused by the autonomic response are very disagreeable and often sickening. The patient develops a fear of the unknown and fear that survival is threatened.

Somatic Pain

The three attributes of somatic pain are a mixture of the attributes of both superficial and visceral pain, although there is no nonvisceral equivalent of visceral colic. Cramps resulting from sustained skeletal muscle contraction are prolonged and may not be intermittent, and the contracted muscles can be palpated. Intestinal or uterine cramps are visceral pains associated with intermittent smooth muscle contraction. Apart from colic any of the attributes of superficial or visceral pain may be found with somatic pain.

REFERRED PAIN

Referred pain is felt in remote areas within the distribution of the same spinal nerve that supplies the site of painful stimulation. Referred pain may be felt in the skin or deeper tissues and is usually well localized; it occurs with moderately severe or severe deep pain and with severe visceral pain. For example, if a balloon is passed into the gallbladder through a cholecystostomy wound and is distended, it causes midline epigastric pain, but as the pain becomes more severe with further distension, the patient also begins to complain of pain in the back at the midline between the scapulae or at the inferior angle of the right scapula. Referred pain may exist in the absence of primary deep pain, but this is very unusual.

When a rarely stimulated structure receives painful stimulation, the pain may be felt at the site of stimulation and also in another area where pain is felt quite frequently. When the pain is felt in another site it is said that the pain is referred from the primary site to the secondary site. It is best understood as a projection of pain to an area commonly the site of past pain. Viscera and other deep structures are uncommon sites for pain; the skin is a common site, so most referred pain is projected from deep structures in the body including the viscera to the surface of the body.

HYPERALGESIA

Within the same spinal segment as a deep pain there may be an increased sensitivity to other stimuli called hyperesthesia. An increased sensitivity to painful stimuli is called hyperalgesia. Primary hyperalgesia is caused by lowering the pain threshold as a result of inflammation, ischemia, nerve injury, or peripheral neuritis. A superficial burning sensation in skin, where the skin appears to be quite normal, should arouse suspicion of damage to a sensory nerve. Local tenderness may be explained by hyperalgesia in deep structures associated with painful deep disease. An area of hyperalgesia is hyperesthetic in the sense that it is more sensitive to most stimuli in the region.

REFLEX MUSCLE CONTRACTION

Skeletal muscles in the same region as an intense deep or visceral pain may undergo stimulation and maintain sustained involuntary contraction. The sustained contraction, a cause for local tenderness in addition to hyperalgesia, can produce pain by itself. Muscle guarding is believed to be a reflex efferent phenomenon just as hyperalgesia is a related afferent phenomenon. Other efferent phenomena may occur, such as smooth muscle contraction and glandular secretion, although they are less easily appreciated. Examples of reflex contraction of skeletal muscles are the rigidity of the abdominal wall muscles with peritonitis, stiff neck with meningeal irritation, and intercostal muscle contraction with severe angina pectoris or severe biliary colic. The muscles involved in rigidity tend to be regional and bilateral rather than unilateral and confined to one spinal segment. Generally muscle guarding occurs only with moderately severe or severe somatic or parietal pain and only with very severe visceral pain.

SUMMARY

Thus there are four types of pain from deep structures in the body; visceral pain arising from viscera only; deep pain, either somatic or parietal, well localized with some characteristics of both visceral and superficial pain; referred pain felt in an area remote from the site of stimulation; and pain from sustained involuntary muscle contraction. Local tenderness may result from regional hyperalgesia or tender muscles in sustained involuntary contraction.

An appreciation of the physiology of pain as it applies to abdominal pain is most helpful in understanding the symptoms and signs of a patient with abdominal pain. Frequently the mechanisms if not the actual diagnosis can be predicted on the basis of the physician's knowledge of the physiology of abdominal pain.

REFERENCES

1. Armstrong D, Jepson JB, Keele CA, Stewart JW: Pain producing substance in human inflammatory exudates and plasma. J Physiol (London) 135:350–370, 1957.
2. Berlin L, Goodell H, Wolff HG: Studies of pain: The relation of pain threshold and pain intensity to the phenomenon of extinction. Trans Am Neurol Assoc: 229–231, 1953.
3. Bigelow N, Harrison I, Goodell H, Wolff HG: Studies on pain: Quantitative measurements of two pain sensations of the skin with reference to the nature of the "hyperalgesia of peripheral neuritis." J Clin Invest 24:503–512, 1945.
4. Catchpole BN: Ileus: Use of sympathetic blocking agents in its treatment. Surgery 66:811–820, 1969.
5. Chapman LF, Ramos A, Goodell H, Silverman G, Wolff HG: A humoral agent implicated in vascular headache of the migraine type. Arch Neurol 3:223–229, 1960.
6. Dworken H, Biel FJ, Machella TE: Supradiaphragmatic reference of pain from the colon. Gastroenterology 22:222–243, 1952.
7. Gasser HS, Erlanger J: The role of fibre size in the establishment of a nerve block by pressure or cocaine. Am J Physiol 88:581–590, 1929.
8. Guyton AC: Textbook of Medical Physiology, 4th ed. Philadelphia: Saunders, 1971.
9. Jones CM: Digestive Tract Pain: Diagnosis and Treatment, Experimental Observations. New York: MacMillan, 1938.
10. Jones CM: Hiatus esophageal hernia. N Engl J Med 225:963–972, 1941.

11. Kuntz A: The Autonomic Nervous System, 4th ed. Philadelphia: Lea & Febiger, 1953.
12. Lewis T: Pain. New York: MacMillan, 1947.
13. Melzack R, Wall PD: Pain mechanisms: A new theory. Science 150:971–979, 1965.
14. Polland WS, Bloomfield AD: Experimental referred pain from the gastrointestinal tract. J Clin Invest 10:435–452, 1931.
15. Ruch TC, Patton HD: Physiology and Biophysics, 19th ed. Philadelphia: Saunders, 1965.
16. Wolff HG, Wolf S: Pain, 2d ed. Springfield, Ill.: Thomas, 1958.

FURTHER READING

Adson AW: Splanchnic pain. Mayo Clin Proc 10:623–624, 1935.

Brooks FP: Gastrointestinal Pathophysiology. London: Oxford, 1974.

Critchley M, O'Leary JL, Jennet B: Scientific Foundations of Neurology. London: Heinemann, 1972.

Haugen FP: The autonomic nervous system and pain. Anesthesiology 29:785–792, 1968.

Jones CM: Pain from the digestive tract. In: Pain, Proceedings of the Association for Research in Nervous and Mental Disease, Dec. 18–19, 1942, New York, pp. 274–288. Baltimore: Williams & Wilkins, 1943.

Kinsella VJ: The Mechanism of Abdominal Pain. Sidney: Australasian, 1948.

Melzack R: The Puzzle of Pain. New York: Basic Books, 1973.

Menaker, GJ: The physiology and mechanism of acute abdominal pain. Surg Clin North Am 42:241–248, 1962.

Chapter 4

Pain Analysis and History Taking

Pain is a symptom; only the sufferer can describe how it feels. The physician should be patient, pay attention to details, and hear the patient out. Ask questions to clarify obscurities—that is history taking. When the main complaint is pain, ask what it was like, where it was felt, when it occurred, how it began, how it subsided, how frequently it occurred, how long it continued, what made it worse, and what made it better—that is pain analysis. Pain is best described by the patient while it is being felt, but it is not always possible for a physician to be present at that time.

There are difficulties in making a diagnosis of pain arising from an internal organ. Several viscera have innervation in common; most have a paucity of sensory nerve endings. Most patients have had little experience with visceral pain. An abdominal pain may arise from a viscus, the walls of a body cavity, a remote area, or muscles undergoing sustained contraction. It can only be described in the patient's own way. Direct questions may be required to determine whether it was superficial or deep, sharp or dull, well or poorly localized, and continuous or intermittent. It is essential to understand what the patient means by such common terms as cramps, gas, burning, aching, and colic.

An accurate and detailed inquiry into various factors related to the pain can lead to an accurate diagnosis in most instances. Early diagnosis is of very great importance in cases of acute pain since urgent management is required and often urgent operation is needed. The ability to recognize the presence or absence of peritonitis, bowel obstruction, or hemorrhage must be mastered.

PAIN ANALYSIS

Normal Pain

Physicians should not forget that some pain is normal; that is, it is not caused by disease or damage. It is generally brief and uncomplicated. For example, transitory precordial discomfort causes anxiety in susceptible individuals particularly if they have a relative or friend with heart disease. The apparent severity varies with the amount of anxiety rather than with the amount of discomfort. A stitch in the side is understood by most people to be a common, uncomfortable sharp pain often made worse by taking a breath. It is believed to be caused by a brief painful contraction of intercostal, abdominal, or diaphragmatic muscle. Pain on moving after a period of rest happens often in old joints. Some limitation of movement in an arthritic joint is to be expected. A sudden severe pain without adequate explanation over an eye is a very uncomfortable sensation, but painful spasm of the frontalis or other nearby muscle must be suspected. Similarly a sharp pain in one ear may be normal. Pain along the whole border of an extremity when there has been no obvious cause is unexplained, and brief periods of transient abdominal pain without aftereffects occur in normal individuals.

Site

The site of a pain, which may also be the point of maximum tenderness, should be located as accurately as possible. This is important in the diagnosis of early appendicitis, Richter's hernia, epigastric hernia, and many other diseases.

Try to decide whether the pain is superficial or deep. For example, a burning sensation along the incision following repair of an inguinal hernia is believed to be caused by damage to either the iliohypogastric or ilioinguinal nerves during operation. The pain and tenderness of pancreatitis is described as deep in the epigastrium. Be aware that the patient may describe a superficial pain as a deep pain because a deep pain may seem more impressive. Sometimes it is more rewarding to ask the patient where it does not hurt rather than where it does hurt. Also decide whether the site of the pain as indicated by the patient is the primary pain, a referred pain, or a pain caused by sustained muscle contraction.

The site of the pain may not indicate the site of disease because several viscera may have the same innervation. The steady visceral pain of diffuse esophageal spasm and angina pectoris are both felt in the center of the chest. A visceral pain felt in the middle of the epigastrium may be the result of disease in any structure derived from the foregut.

Extent

The size of the area where the pain is felt has some importance in diagnosis. Although the rash of herpes zoster may be quite limited in extent, the associated pain is felt in almost the whole distribution of the spinal or cranial nerve involved. The pain of active duodenal ulcer disease is limited to a small area, whereas the pain of acute gastroenteritis or diffuse peritonitis is felt over the whole abdomen.

Localization varies with the density of the nerve endings and is therefore more precise in the skin than in deeper structures. The site where the diffuse pain began should be determined. In many cases of diffuse peritonitis the patient can give a history of the pain's beginning in one part of the abdomen, and this is an important clue to the cause of the peritonitis. Prior to the widespread pain of acute peritonitis the abdominal pain is localized in the right lower quadrant in perforated appendicitis, the left lower quadrant in perforated diverticulitis, the right upper quadrant in perforated cholecystitis, and in the epigastrium in perforated duodenal ulcer. The pain of widespread peritoneal irritation may have begun in the lower abdomen as in bleeding from an ectopic pregnancy or in the left upper quadrant as in rupture of the spleen.

A widespread pain may become localized. For example, in acute appendicitis the poorly localized periumbilical pain later becomes localized to McBurney's point. In acute appendicitis the initial periumbilical steady or crampy pain is a visceral pain resulting from irritation of the midgut. The pain disappears as parietal pain develops in the region of the inflamed appendix when the inflammation reaches the parietal peritoneum. Localization is more precise with pleural or parietal peritoneal than with visceral pain.

Primary Pain

It may be difficult to differentiate a primary pain from a referred pain. A midline visceral pain is often the first pain felt in disease of the gastrointestinal tract, and pain at the site of the disease begins later as inflammation irritates the nearby parietal peritoneum. For example, biliary colic is a visceral pain felt in the midline of the epigastrium. Later, when inflammation of the gallbladder becomes established, a parietal pain occurs at the site of the gallbladder in the right upper quadrant. This pain may be associated with yet a third pain, a referred pain in the back at the inferior angle of the right scapula.

Referred Pain

A deep pain is often but not necessarily associated with a referred pain. Referred pain may occur rarely in the absence of a primary pain at the site of irritation and remains in the same spinal segment as the primary pain. If the irritation is intense, spread may occur proximally to the next spinal nerve or in the same nerve segment on the other side of the body. When pain occurs and the site of the disease is not clear, study the site and extent of the pain and then consider the entire distribution of that spinal nerve. In this way all likely sources of pain come under scrutiny. Classic examples of referred pain of diagnostic significance are shoulder top (not tip) pain with irritation of the central diaphragm (C4), pain along the inner side of the left forearm (T1) and left arm (T2) with severe angina pectoris, pain at the inferior angle of the right scapula with acute cholecystitis (T8), and pain in the groin and genital area with ureteral colic (L1). Referred pain from lesions in the distribution of the second or lower lumbar spinal nerves is not felt as abdominal pain because these segments supply the back, the lower limb, and the pelvis. Muscle rigidity is poorly localized in that it often tends to involve a group of muscles on both sides of the body.

Circumstances at Onset

Ask the patient if anyone else has a similar pain that began at the same time. Other persons at the table who ate the same contaminated food may have nausea and vomiting, crampy abdominal pain, and diarrhea simultaneously. Pain following endoscopic examinations or an enema should immediately make one suspect injury and possible perforation.

Heartburn appearing only on recumbency, straining, or stooping is typical of a lax lower esophageal sphincter allowing reflux of gastric contents into the lower esophagus. Back pain or upper abdominal pain that appears while the patient is standing an hour or so after drinking fluids but that is relieved soon after lying down suggests poor drainage from the renal pelvis. Pain on straining, sneezing, or coughing may indicate an inguinal hernia if the pain occurs in the inguinal canal or nerve root pressure if it occurs in the spinal region or in the distribution of an appropriate spinal nerve.

Crampy abdominal pain in the hypogastrium followed by diarrhea may occur in any condition with rapid intestinal transit. Urgency to open the bowels is a frequent accompaniment. Tenesmus, a painful persistent desire to empty the bowel, occurs as a complication of a regional painful disease such as prostatitis, cervicitis, inflamed hemorrhoids, or infiltrating tumor low in the pelvis. Acute tearing pain during defecation is caused by anal fissure. Pain after bowel movement may be caused either by fissure or congested hemorrhoids. Abdominal pain after straining may be caused by renewed enlargement of an abdominal aneurysm.

If after eating or drinking a large amount the patient vomits, immediately complains of chest pain, and collapses, one must suspect spontaneous rupture of the esophagus. Pain that follows drinking alcoholic beverages must be suspected of being caused by gastritis, pancreatitis, peptic ulcer, or esophagitis.

A clear statement of what the patient was doing at the onset of the pain can be important. Did the pain follow an injury? An injury to the left upper abdomen, left flank, or left lower chest even months before is significant if delayed rupture of the spleen is a possibility. Was the patient asleep? Any pain that awakens a patient from sleep is very likely to be important and usually has an organic rather than a psychogenic cause. Did the patient take a laxative? Cramps followed by diarrhea are expected after a laxative, but cramps without diarrhea may indicate an obstruction. A worsening right lower quadrant abdominal pain after a purgative may be caused by aggravated acute appendicitis. Is the patient diabetic, and if so, is the diabetes in control? Abdominal pain in an uncontrolled diabetic is bizarre yet is only a problem if diabetic acidosis is not diagnosed or is forgotten as a cause for abdominal pain. Control of diabetes mellitus coincides with disappearance of this poorly understood abdominal pain.

Precipitating Factors

A precipitating factor is one that appears to lead directly to the onset of the pain, whereas an aggravating factor is one that makes a pain worse and causes it to persist. From the practical point of view the two overlap, and the differentiation is not very important. Evening or nighttime pain following a fatty meal is a frequent history with biliary colic. Pain during swallowing suggests an esophageal spasm, stenosis, peptic ulcer, or carcinoma of the esophagus. Pain on going to work, on meeting people, or while involved in an unappealing activity done in unpleasant surroundings is a conversion symptom. The anxious patient may be a poor sleeper and may complain of early morning distress. If he or she complains of always being tired on awakening, a psychogenic problem is likely. It is better to recognize the hysteric or neurotic patient early and then give the added confidence of obvious recognition, thus avoiding numerous negative tests and X-rays. On the other hand an anxious patient with cancerphobia may only be satisfied after radiological investigations are reported negative. Anxiety, depression, or other emotional disturbances are frequent precipitating factors in psychogenic pain.

Time of Day, Month, Season

Pain made worse by physical and mental activity is present during the daytime while the patient is alert and active. For this reason locomotive, digestive, eye, and psychogenic pains tend to be daytime rather than nighttime problems. Sinus pain may be bothersome first thing in the morning because of poor drainage during the night. Rheumatoid arthritic joints are painful at the beginning of movement after a period of rest, whereas osteoarthritic joints become painful with use or immediately afterward. The pain of irritable colon syndrome starts early in the morning, whereas the pain of peptic ulcer rarely begins before breakfast.

Peptic ulcer pain, especially from a duodenal ulcer, tends to occur several hours after breakfast, at midmorning coffee time, just before lunch, several hours after lunch, immediately before supper, a few hours after supper, and during the night. It tends to be troublesome for several weeks or months then disappears for weeks or months. There is an unexplained tendency to recurrence in the spring and the fall.

Night pain, especially if it is the cause of the patient's awakening, is significant and usually indicates organic disease. Sleep allows increased autonomic activity so that the pain of peptic ulcer and crampy pain may be bothersome at night. The pain of rheumatic or tuberculous bone or joint disease may be aggravated during the night because of relaxation of protective muscle guarding. Burning retrosternal pain when first lying down is typical of heartburn caused by esophageal reflux. The constant steady pain of an infiltrating tumor may be more troublesome once the day's distractions cease. Psychogenic pain may be troublesome at night if the individual has insomnia.

Lower abdominal pain occurring two weeks before an expected period may be caused by bleeding at ovulation. (Since the conventional contraceptive pill generally suppresses ovulation, pain from such bleeding is unlikely to occur.) A venereal infection can become established more readily during menstruation than at other times, and therefore acute salpingitis occurs more frequently soon after menstruation than at other times in the menstrual cycle.

Sinus congestion pain is expected to be seasonal if the related allergies are seasonal. Chest pain resulting from respiratory infections is most frequent in cold weather. Joint pain is worse in damp, cool weather. Intestinal cramps from oxalic acid in green apples are most common before the harvest.

Mode and Speed of Onset

The type of onset, whether gradual or sudden, and the rapidity of progression may provide useful information in making the diagnosis. Apart from an injury, abrupt or sudden onset of abdominal pain suggests a mechanical cause, which almost always requires urgent surgical care. Perforation of a viscus, hemorrhage, embolism, and torsion of a viscus are examples of painful complications having very sudden onset.

Rapid onset suggests a brief period during which the patient realizes that the pain is becoming rapidly worse. The pain of intestinal obstruction, ureteral obstruction, mesenteric vascular thrombosis, biliary colic, and acute pancreatitis develops over a brief period of time. Abdominal inflammations, infiltrations by malignant tumors, and metabolic diseases develop more slowly. The pain of malignant tumor growth is often limited but relentless. The patient may have difficulty remembering the time of onset if very slow, and if an obstruction develops quite slowly there may be no pain. For example, massive distension of the bile ducts and gallbladder can occur painlessly if obstruction develops slowly, such as by a growth at the duodenal papilla. The slow onset of pain with limited discomfort may result in a delay in seeking medical attention.

Quality and Character

If there were specific nerve endings for each type of pain, patients would be able to report reliably the characteristic symptoms, and diagnosis would be simple. Unfortunately the patient's description of the quality of the pain is not helpful other than to understand its constancy or intermittency. The quality of the pain is unlikely to be the most important factor in making a diagnosis. There are a few types of pain that are characteristic, such as the burning pain of peptic ulcer and esophagitis, the tearing pain of dissecting aneurysm and anal fissure, the squeezing tightness of angina pectoris and biliary colic, the pounding pain of aneurysmal erosion of bone, and the lightning pain of tabes dorsalis.

Imagination tends to make patients' descriptions vary widely. To help identify the nature of the pain try to relate the description to the time-intensity curves. It is necessary to decide whether the patient is complaining of a superficial, deep, or visceral pain. Is it sharp or dull? If the pain arises from deep structures, is it a well localized clear somatic pain, or a poorly localized midline visceral pain? Do not go further into the patient's description of the quality or character of the pain. It is more rewarding to spend more time on pain analysis than to listen to the patient's attempt to describe the quality of the pain. Always remember that the patient's need to impress may be unintentionally misleading.

Change in Quality and Character

Although identification of the character of an abdominal pain is important, it is perhaps more important to recognize a change in character. At the onset there may be a midline poorly localized visceral pain. Remember that a visceral pain, either steady or crampy, may be only the first of several types of pain. By its location it indicates the embryologic section of the gastrointestinal tract to which the affected organ belongs and perhaps suggests the possible mechanism. Steady visceral pain suggests increasing distension or ischemia whereas crampy pain indicates exaggerated intestinal activity. Every patient having visceral pain which is likely to change with time, must be examined repeatedly. Inflammation may occur causing parietal pain to begin as visceral pain disappears, a very significant change. The classic example is the steady or crampy periumbilical pain that changes to the well-localized pain of acute appendicitis at McBurney's point in the right lower quadrant of the abdomen.

Further changes may occur in the quality and character of pain. A somatic or parietal pain may give rise to a referred pain. The inflamed organ may rupture changing a localized pain into the widespread abdominal pain of diffuse peritonitis. Referred pain might follow. A typical sequence begins with gallstones causing obstruction resulting in biliary colic (a visceral pain), which changes to acute cholecystitis (a somatic pain) associated with pain at the inferior angle of the right scapula (a referred pain). As the pathological changes worsen empyema, gangrene, and perforation with diffuse peritonitis (a diffuse parietal pain) follow and right shoulder top pain (another referred pain) occurs.

It cannot be too strongly emphasized that the patient with undiagnosed abdominal pain demands repeated examinations because of possible changes in the quality and location of the pain, the probability of associated symptoms appearing, and changes in the abdominal physical signs, any of which may be diagnostic.

Intensity or Severity

Evaluation of the severity of abdominal pain is difficult. Try to assess the psychic reaction and compare that with what should be expected according to the patient's cultural background, training, age, the severity of other signs of illness, the severity of the physiological reactions to pain, and the patient's attitude. The patient's personality, past experience, and emotional balance are difficult to evaluate quickly during a brief interview.

Mothers often compare the new pain to labor–pain in childbirth varies from delivery to delivery as well as among mothers. Previously injured men relate the severity of the new pain to the severity of their previous experiences. The severity of pain may be grossly misinterpreted in the elderly, the debilitated, the acutely ill, and the severely injured.

The most severe abdominal pains include renal colic, perforated duodenal ulcer, acute hemorrhagic pancreatitis, small bowel obstruction, biliary colic, mesenteric vascular occlusion, strangulated hernia, and dissecting aortic aneurysm. Almost every abdominal pain that is severe and lasts longer than 6 hours is likely to be serious and to require urgent surgical management. Secondary shock with pain is extremely serious.

When the pain is less severe, try to determine how much the pain appears to interfere with work, play, and sleep. Some indication of severity is given by a history of remaining upright, lying down, falling down, fainting, crying out, or groaning. Inquire into the measures taken to obtain relief. Note especially the dosage of any analgesic taken and its effects. Broadly speaking the severity of a pain indicates its importance. It may be more accurate to deduce the severity of pain from the success of pain relief by various measures including drugs rather than by attempting to assess the severity from the symptoms and signs of the physiological reactions to the pain.

Frequency

The frequency, duration, and character of the pain are determined by the mode of production. A good example of frequently recurring pain is the pain of active duodenal ulcer. Biliary colic rarely recurs in a 24-hour period. The frequency of recurrences within the day, week, month, or year may be significant for diagnosis and may give an indication of severity. Angina pectoris may occur several times within an hour. Acute pancreatitis is unlikely to recur within 24 hours.

Duration and Course

The speed of onset, the rapidity of culmination, the duration and smoothness of maximal pain, and the rapidity of regression of pain provide important clues to the diagnosis of abdominal pain. Persisting severe pain is unusual since nerve endings fatigue, defense mechanisms break down, infection develops, and shock appears. Even with less severe pain, constancy is unusual; when this is claimed, one might consider psychogenic pain. Several exceptions to this general rule are causalgia, phantom limb pain, herpes zoster, skeletal metastases, and carcinoma of a viscus such as the pancreas.

The course of pain may suggest its cause. A steady, relentless deep aching pain in the epigastrium suggests pancreatic carcinoma. A throbbing pain is an intermittent somatic pain because of the pulse. A frequent cause of throbbing pain is abscess. Each wave of intestinal colic lasts less than 5 minutes. Biliary and renal colic persist for at least 15 minutes; generally they last between $\frac{1}{2}$ and 4 hours. If a pain originally thought to be biliary colic lasts longer than 6 hours, then the diagnosis of acute cholecystitis is justified since inflammation has supervened. Angina pectoris lasts for only a few minutes. If angina does not subside within 20 minutes, there is strong suspicion of myocardial infarction. Similarly when angina does not disappear within several minutes after taking nitroglycerin, the diagnosis of uncomplicated angina is in doubt.

The mode of decline of pain may help indicate the cause. Rapid improvement suggests release of a blockage or prompt response to treatment by antacid, antispasmodic, or narcotic. The apparent improvement of the pain of acute appendicitis or acute cholecystitis may be deceptive since it may be soon followed by diffuse peritonitis resulting from rupture of an empyema of the appendix or gallbladder.

Aggravating Factors

Most abdominal pain is intensified by certain specific factors that are of importance. Relief may be obtained by removing an aggravating factor or by applying an opposing (relieving) factor, both of which have diagnostic significance. Anticipation of food or delay in taking food causes aggravation of the pain of peptic ulcer. Appealing, tasty foods, including sweets, increase gastric acid secretion. Irritants such as hot and cold foods, spices, acids, and alcoholic fluids increase gastric acidity and aggravate the pain of peptic ulcer, gastritis, and reflux esophagitis. Fat delays gastric emptying and the onset of pain after meals. Food roughage is said to increase the pain of peptic ulcer. Peptic ulcer pain is aggravated several hours after eating when gastric acid is unbuffered, because food has left the stomach. Emotional stress increases the severity, duration, and frequency of the pain of duodenal ulcer.

Obesity, straining, lying flat, or stooping increases intra-abdominal pressure and gastroesophageal reflux in patients with incompetent lower esophageal sphincter; reflux of acid gastric juice results in heartburn. Fatty foods stimulate the gallbladder to contract and may precipitate or aggravate biliary colic. Protein stimulates pancreatic secretion; so protein foods may exacerbate the pain of pancreatitis. Foods or alcoholic beverages tend to aggravate pancreatitis regardless of its cause. Eating stimulates the gastrocolic reflex, which in turn stimulates the lower intestine; the pain of many lower bowel disorders is intensified by eating. Intestinal angina is precipitated or aggravated by eating because digestion increases the need for splanchnic blood flow on an impaired splanchnic circulation.

Abdominal pain after eating may have a variety of causes. Activity after a meal, cold, and emotional distress aggravate angina pectoris. Lactose-containing dairy products cause the bloating, cramps, and diarrhea in lactase-deficient individuals. As a rule abdominal distress within a few minutes of eating is caused by gastric distension. Abdominal swelling, especially after meals, may result from excessive air swallowing. Deep lower thoracic or epigastric pain appearing with exercise suggests angina pectoris.

Pain initiated by movement and relieved by rest is typical of a musculoskeletal disorder. The pain of an abdominal inflammatory process is aggravated by movement. Pain aggravated by coughing or sneezing suggests peritoneal irritation or nerve root pressure caused by an intraspinal lesion. Steady epigastric pain made worse by lying supine suggests pancreatic disease. A patient with abdominal cramps does not choose to lie supine and immobile but moves about during the colic. Pain made worse by voiding suggests a genitourinary lesion.

Pain aggravated by breathing suggests pleuritic pain or a lesion just below the diaphragm. The pain disappears if the breath is held in expiration but if the breath is held in inspiration the intra-abdominal lesion may remain painful because of increased pressure from the contracted diaphragm.

Relieving Factors

Relieving factors are often the opposite of aggravating factors, although there are some that have no opposite action.

Fasting does not relieve but aggravates the distress of peptic ulcer; food that is bland, soft, uninteresting, and nonstimulating tends to relieve peptic ulcer pain. Peptic ulcer pain is best controlled by food and antacid medication. Spices, acids, and alcoholic beverages are forbidden for peptic ulcer patients, but milk is widely used by patients to relieve the pain. Protein buffers acid; yet amino acids are a stimulus for gastric secretion. Emotional balance and relief from stress are most important in control of duodenal ulcer disease.

The time taken to feel relief from burning pain after swallowing an antacid is of great diagnostic importance. Immediate relief on swallowing a liquid antacid localizes the site of irritation to the lower esophagus. In fact reflux esophagitis pain is immediately relieved by taking milk, fats, and oils and by swallowing air. Relief within 5 to 10 minutes is expected in most patients with gastric or stomal ulcer. Relief of the distress of duodenal ulcer disease takes 7 to 15 minutes following antacid ingestion. Relief beginning more than 30 minutes after antacid ingestion is rarely the result of the antacid.

Reducing body weight, avoiding tight clothing, eating frequent small meals, using a bland ulcer diet, avoiding stooping, and elevating the head of the bed reduces gastroesophageal reflux and thereby prevents heartburn and esophagitis. Avoiding fatty foods does not relieve biliary colic but may prevent some attacks. The only satisfactory method of resting the pancreas to allow pancreatitis to subside is continuous gastric suction.

Because eating generally stimulates the gastrointestinal tract, avoiding food affords some relief in painful lower intestinal disorders. The cramps of partial small bowel obstruction in Crohn's disease improve with starvation. Cramps from steatorrhea do not occur if fats are eliminated. When lactase-deficient individuals avoid lactose-containing dairy products the abdominal bloating, cramps, and diarrhea disappear.

Early postprandial distress from air swallowing is relieved by belching. As a rule the gas-prone individual swallows air repeatedly and publicly displays the gas problem. Vomiting affords relief when the stomach is overdistended by food or fluid. For those with progressive pyloric narrowing from long-standing duodenal ulcer disease evening vomiting becomes a regular event.

Pain from lesions in the lower bowel is relieved by a bowel movement as a general rule. Urgent defecation followed by relief of periumbilical visceral pain is frequent in patients having regional ileitis. Unplugging a colonic obstruction by enemas or intubating a sigmoid volvulus affords immediate relief with the passage of much flatus and liquid feces.

Musculoskeletal and other somatic pains are less severe during rest since movement causes pain. Similarly the pain of inflammatory disease in the abdomen is not aggravated if the patient remains immobile and supine and breathes shallowly. Patients with colic writhe and often assume a flexed posture since drawing the knees up against the abdomen appears to afford some relief. The patient with pancreatic pain may sit forward and support the epigastrium for relief; preference for this position is more typical of pancreatic carcinoma than pancreatitis.

Patients for whom breathing is painful breathe shallowly, and are frightened of coughing or sneezing because both cause sudden increases in pain. Pleuritic pain is relieved as a pleural effusion develops separating parietal and visceral pleuras. Occasionally one may notice relief of a hepatic or splenic friction rub as ascitic fluid separates the membranes, or adhesions develop that fix the viscus to the parietal peritoneum.

Heat applied to a painful area promotes muscle relaxation and gives relief if the pain is the result of smooth or skeletal muscle contraction. Heat may increase pain in an inflammation by irritating an area already hyperalgesic by increasing vascularity and by increasing tissue fluid pressure and edema. In spite of this, moderate heat helps to localize infection.

Finally a warning with regard to pain relief in abdominal disorders is repeated. Temporary relief may not mean improvement but may be followed shortly by worsening of the patient's condition. Classic examples are the temporary relief of local pain on rupture of an empyema of the appendix or gallbladder, rupture of an acute paracolic diverticular abscess, or rupture of other intra-abdominal abscess into the peritoneal cavity. The relief of pain is temporary and soon followed by severe acute peritonitis with the threat of septic shock and death.

Accompanying Symptoms

Many symptoms that accompany abdominal pain are important in pain analysis while others are so nonspecific that they contribute little. The presence of some symptoms aids in the appreciation of the severity of the illness or the onset of complications rather than the severity of the abdominal pain.

Appetite is a conditioned reflex that can be stimulated by smell, sight, or even the memory of appealing food. Hunger is a primitive unconditioned physiological state resulting from the deprivation of food. Anorexia is a lack of desire for food, and generally means absence of both appetite and hunger. Anorexia has many causes including emotional upset, drugs, metabolic changes, vascular changes, and many diseases.

Nausea is a feeling of revulsion for food, is largely of central origin, and in abdominal diseases is followed in many instances by vomiting. Vomiting without nausea occurs in many central nervous system diseases. Nausea is usually accompanied by autonomic vasomotor and secretory reactions, such as faintness, weakness, sweating, pallor, and palpitations. Gastric hypotonicity, reversed peristalsis, and gastric dilatation are accompaniments. Distension of the lower esophagus and irritation of the oropharynx are potent stimuli for vomiting.

Fainting may indicate a severe pain. If a stoic individual is forced to leave work or take to bed because of pain, it can be assumed to be severe. A call for help from a patient who rarely calls is more likely to be important than a call from a patient who complains incessantly.

Accompanying Signs

Pain analysis consists of history taking in such detail that the provisional diagnosis is often the correct diagnosis. In this section the signs referred to are those from the history given by the patient or observed by others rather than physical signs found by the physician on clinical examination.

Vomiting is preceded by anorexia and nausea in most instances except in diseases of the central nervous system. Most visceral diseases when severe and accompanied by massive visceral afferent stimulation, such as major trauma, infection, obstruction, or perforation, are accompanied by vomiting. There are many causes other than abdominal disease, but the emphasis in this section is on the conditions associated with abdominal disease. Nausea and vomiting occur readily in children with gastroenteritis, in alcoholics, and in adults with peptic ulcer disease. An undilated obstructed esophagus causes regurgitation of every few swallows, and the regurgitated material consists of masticated food mixed with saliva only. Large volumes of vomitus from the esophagus indicate esophageal dilatation, and esophageal dilatation is most commonly associated with achalasia.

Pyloric obstruction, with which the stomach is greatly distended, causes vomiting of large volumes. If the stomach is infiltrated and rigid, distension does not occur and vomiting is more frequent and smaller in volume. The dilated stomach with complete pyloric obstruction holds all food and fluids taken that day. The large vomitus may contain recognizable vegetable matter eaten several meals prior to the vomiting. The vomitus does not contain bile when the pylorus is completely occluded. The patient becomes dehydrated and develops an electrolyte imbalance leading to metabolic alkalosis. Vomiting food eaten at previous meals means gastric stasis, and large volume vomiting means gorging, stasis, or pyloric obstruction. If bile is seen in the vomitus it shows that the pylorus and bile ducts are open. Pyloric reflux of bile is normal. If the color of vomitus changes from yellow-green to orange it suggests low small intestinal obstruction.

Bleeding is always investigated since it may be serious. Bleeding from varices in the lower esophagus is usually bright red. If the gastric contents are acidic, liquid blood develops small brown clots resembling coffee grounds. When the bleeding is massive, pure blood is vomited. Unchanged blood of less than massive quantities indicates ulceration in an achlorhydric stomach, suggesting gastric carcinoma.

Regurgitation of every swallow suggests a high esophageal obstruction, whereas vomiting of sour or bitter food indicates a lesion below the esophagus. Early and frequent vomiting occurs in small bowel obstruction. Low small bowel obstruction may cause periumbilical cramps first, then distension and vomiting. Colonic obstruction causes abdominal distension early followed by vomiting later.

Toxic vomiting complicates pancreatitis, gastritis, peritonitis with advanced ileus, and high small bowel obstruction. Toxic vomiting is said to be reflex because it is active and forceful. Persistent toxic vomiting is associated with much retching. Regurgitant or reflux vomiting occurs in paralytic ileus and low colonic obstruction when there is also passive welling up of contents of the overfilled intestinal tract with effortless vomiting. In the elderly or in others with depressed pharyngeal and laryngeal reflexes there is great danger of pulmonary aspiration. Typical projectile vomiting occurs in infants with hypertrophic pyloric stenosis only, if one considers projectile vomiting as long-range vomiting in relation to the patient's size.

Diarrhea occurs with enteritis and colitis and with inflammation in the pelvis, such as pelvic abscess, pelvic inflammatory disease, and proctitis. A pelvic inflammation is associated with cramps, tenesmus, and increased mucus secretion into the rectum causing a mucus diarrhea. Frequent hypogastric cramps and bloody diarrhea suggest chronic ulcerative colitis. Incomplete rectal obstruction by a large fecal mass may cause paradoxical spurious diarrhea in which case odorous diarrhea and hard fecal masses on rectal examination are found. Fecal impaction occurs in the aged, in infants, and in adults taking constipating analgesics without laxatives. Constipation may cause crampy abdominal pain because of obstruction at stenosing lesions or at fresh surgical anastomoses or because of impaction of feces in the rectum.

Bleeding may be an important sign in the diagnosis of abdominal pain. Rapid transit may allow bright red blood to appear in the stools from bleeding into the stomach. As a rule bleeding from the small bowel or higher is changed to melena, a shiny, tarry black stool having a characteristic odor. Bleeding from the right colon might be bright red or dark red depending upon the frequency of bowel movements.

Blood in the urine indicates problems with the kidneys or other urinary organs. Jaundice with abdominal pain directs attention to the bile ducts and pancreas or, if there is hemolysis and anemia, to the spleen. Gaseous distension of the abdomen is an accompaniment of both mechanical and paralytic intestinal obstruction. Bloating with diarrhea and crampy abdominal pain suggests incomplete intestinal obstruction. Gaseous distension is not a feature of gastroenteritis or colitis unless toxic megacolon develops. Toxic megacolon is a serious and dangerous complication of colitis.

Attitude and Behavior

The more dramatic and detailed but vague the description of pain, the greater the possibility of major psychological disturbances and the greater the possibility of psychogenic pain. The mechanism and motivation may be deeply hidden so that the patient does not appreciate that the pain has a subconscious origin and that there are subconscious aims to gain some gratification through complaining. The neurotic is unaware of this motivation; the malingerer is deliberately attempting to deceive.

Responses to Therapy

The patient in pain may be treated by analgesics or other measures directed to pain relief only, but most patients are managed more appropriately by treatment of the abnormality causing the pain. Most patients remember measures that were previously effective in relieving pain but some may recall the success of the treatment only on direct questioning. Patients tend to discount partially successful therapy and may consider the degree of relief too unimportant to have mentioned it in describing relieving factors during pain analysis.

Occasionally a pain is duplicated during an examination. Distension of the colon during sigmoidoscopy or while receiving an enema may initiate cramps in an irritable or spastic colon. Examination for movement at a joint may cause a musculoskeletal pain to reappear. Local pressure may elicit tenderness similar to the original pain. A trial of therapy may be important in pain analysis for diagnosis. When the patient complains of colic yet the physician doubts its presence, an injection of a potent antispasmodic may clearly decide who is correct. When a patient complains of a steady pain and demands injections for relief yet the physician doubts that the patient has such pain, relief with a placebo injection of saline suggests but does not prove that the physician is correct.

HISTORY TAKING

In essence pain analysis is a precise and detailed history of the patient's pain. Features of the patient's medical history other than pain analysis include age; sex; geographic regions during birth, childhood, and adult life; functional inquiry; past health; family history; and personal history.

Age

History taking from children is sometimes difficult and often misleading because of the child's immaturity and the parents' natural tendency to interpret features of the child's illness rather than to report their observations objectively. Parents may have all of the difficulties of patients in addition to the obvious difficulty of having no personal experience with their child's pain.

Under the age of 2 years the major cause for serious abdominal pain is intussusception. Primary intussusception is rare beyond the age of 3 years, after which intussusception is almost invariably secondary to a local lesion of the bowel. Acute appendicitis is rare under the age of 2 years but may occur at any other age. Malignant disease of the gastrointestinal tract and pancreatitis unrelated to gallstones occurs with increasing frequency beyond the age of 25 years. The complications of diverticular disease of the colon, gallstones, and cardiovascular disease increase in frequency with age.

Sex

Acquired diseases related to the sex organs occur after sexual maturity. Carcinoma of the prostate and benign prostatic hypertrophy occur with increasing frequency as males grow older. During the reproductive period, all of the abnormalities of organs related to childbearing take place, such as intraperitoneal bleeding with ovulation, complications of pregnancy, endometriosis, and diseases of the fallopian tubes. After the menarche most diseases of the uterus and ovaries increase in frequency with age. Uterine fibroids rarely develop after the menopause.

Geographic Regions

The geographic districts where the patient was born and has lived have a bearing on the likelihood of disease. Some diseases are more common to regions because of climate, environmental conditions, or the racial characteristics of the people who are native to the area. Some diseases occur with equal frequency in all peoples living in a region, whereas other diseases are restricted to those of similar racial background. Environmental factors, especially infections and infestations, may cause disease in visitors to endemic areas. Often the disease contracted by visitors is more serious than the same disease in natives. Contact with visitors from areas of endemic disease should be noted.

Functional Inquiry

Functional inquiry is a search for symptoms by surveying the functions of all body systems. Symptoms directly related to the chief complaint appear in the history of present illness. The efficiency with which significant symptoms related to the present illness are included in its history rather than in the functional inquiry is a measure of the physician's experience and ability. When the diagnosis is obscure, the functional inquiry should be taken and recorded in greatest detail.

Past Health

The history of past health should be determined as accurately as possible. There should be a detailed chronological record of all illnesses, operations, and injuries with their outcomes. There should be specific inquiry regarding diseases that might have caused permanent or progressive damage, such as rheumatic fever, tuberculosis, nephritis, hepatitis, or diabetes mellitus. Special note should be made of those diseases prone to recurrence, such as malignant neoplasms, peptic ulcer, alcoholism, pancreatitis, tuberculosis, Crohn's disease, and ulcerative colitis. An accurate list of all medications taken recently, continuously, or frequently must be made; iatrogenic illnesses are not uncommon.

All operations should be noted with as much accuracy as possible and should include the reason for the operation, the operation performed, the complications, and the results. It might be very important to know whether an incidental appendectomy had been performed as part of an unrelated operation in the region. Intraperitoneal adhesions are responsible for bowel obstruction more commonly after operations in the lower abdomen and pelvis than in the upper abdomen. Adhesions rarely cause complications other than complete or intermittent bowel obstruction. A detailed listing of injuries both physical and chemical is important. Alcohol often causes damage to the liver, pancreas, stomach, or brain.

Family History

Detailed inquiry should be made into any physical or mental health problems in parents, siblings, and close relatives. Those diseases having familial predisposition should receive special attention. Inherited traits and diseases are restricted to blood relatives, whereas infectious diseases can affect those who have joined the family by marriage.

Personal History

An inquiry is made into the patient's place of birth, childhood, schooling, and occupation. The attitude of the patient to his or her parents, siblings, friends, and work associates is sought. The marital record should include a notation concerning compatibility of the partners, domestic arrangements, and living conditions. The patient's worries should be remarked whether related to health, social, or financial problems. Personal habits are noted, especially those related to medications, smoking, alcohol drinking, exercise, and hobbies. The patient's apparent reaction to stress is observed.

HISTORY-TAKING DIFFICULTIES

While the clinician is taking the history of the abdominal pain from the patient, there are at least five steps each of which is open to error. First, the clinician must formulate the question. Next, the patient must interpret the clinician's question and relate this to the perceived abdominal pain. The patient then tries to describe the sensation. The examiner listens to the patient's description and tries to understand what is intended by the words and expressions used. Finally the physician analyzes symptoms and unravels their meanings as well as possible.

The problems in taking a history become more complex if a translator is needed. The translator may err in interpreting the clinician's question and/or the patient's story. The result is the translator's version of the patient's history. The physician has the added task of trying to determine what the translator has interpreted.

As a rule the first 5 minutes of the patient's story are the most important. Simply listen and pay attention. Almost everything that the patient feels is of greatest importance is said first. The patient's choice of words and expressions may reveal anxiety or fear, attitudes toward the illness, personality characteristics, and reaction to pain. The physician must then ask questions to confirm important facts. For example, the physician should not accept the patient's word that a colic or cramp was felt. The patient may not understand the medical meaning of these words or may have chosen these words to impress the physician with the importance or severity of the pain. The clinician may be obliged to ask direct questions to ascertain with certainty the patient's meanings, but leading questions should be kept to a minimum.

When history taking is difficult or there appears to be a problem in understanding the patient, it may be wise to plan a second visit for a review of this history. On the second occasion the patient will have reconsidered the description and a second try may be an improvement. In the interval the patient will have consulted his or her spouse or parents. Haste in investigating before an accurate history is taken may result in excessive investigation. Remember that laboratory data can be faulty and X-ray appearances may be suggestive but not diagnostic. Superfluous investigation may in itself promote anxiety.

If the physician believes an accurate history has been taken yet the symptoms are unreasonable for organic illness, psychogenic pain should be considered. The diagnosis of psychogenic pain should not be entirely based on exclusion of organic disease. Symptoms tend to be grossly exaggerated by the neurotic, but these embellishments are easily recognized. If the patient denies relief from the use of strong analgesics, the history varies on repeated questioning, or the patient appears to be quite indifferent to disabling symptoms or totally incapacitated from minor symptoms, be alert to the possibility of a neurotic, a hypochondriac, a malingerer, or a narcotic addict. The neurotic or hypochondriac patient does not know that the apparent illness has something other than an organic cause; the malingerer knows that he or she is well yet tries to deceive. The addict feigns illness in order to obtain narcotics.

The accuracy of the history of abdominal pain can be improved by reviewing the symptoms with the patient on several occasions. It may be wise to interview the patient's spouse, relatives, or previous physicians. Medical records departments of hospitals where the patient has been treated should be asked for clinical summaries. If information from these sources is consistent, the accuracy of the history should be accepted.

The aim of history taking is to elicit and record as much information as possible that might be helpful in making the diagnosis. In most cases of abdominal pain the diagnosis is made from pain analysis. After determining the apparent depth of the pain and its constancy, diagnosis will come from answers to the questions beginning with what, where, when, how, how often, how long, what aggravates, and what relieves.

FURTHER READING

Boles ET, Zollinger RM: The acute abdomen–medical aspects. Med Clin North Am 40:499–512, 1956.

Botsford TW, Wilson RE: The Acute Abdomen, 2d ed. Philadelphia: Saunders, 1977.

Cope Z: The Early Diagnosis of the Acute Abdomen, 14th ed. London: Oxford, 1972.

Farmer DA: Abdominal pain. Med Clin North Am 41:1287–1302, 1957.

Gelin L, Nyhus LM, Condon RE: Abdominal Pain. Philadelphia: Lippincott, 1969.

Harvey AB, Bordley J: Differential Diagnosis, 2d ed. Philadelphia: Saunders, 1970.

Heffernon EW, Reaves LE III: Consideration in the diagnosis of abdominal pain. Med Clin North Am 50:439–447, 1966.

Janzen R, editor: Pain Analysis. Bristol: Wright, 1970.

Jones CM: Pain from the digestive tract. In: Pain, Proceedings of the Association for Research in Nervous and Mental Disease, Dec. 18–19, 1942, New York, pp. 274–288. Baltimore: Williams & Wilkins, 1943.

Jones PF: Emergency Abdominal Surgery in Infancy, Childhood, and Adult Life. Oxford: Blackwell, 1974.

MacBryde CM: Signs and Symptoms, 5th ed. Philadelphia: Lippincott, 1970.

Mellinkoff SM: The Differential Diagnosis of Abdominal Pain. New York: McGraw-Hill, 1959.

Menaker GJ: The physiology and mechanisms of acute abdominal pain. Surg Clin North Am 42:241–248, 1962.

Moore SW: The physiological basis for diagnostic signs of an acute abdomen. Surg Clin North Am 38:371–383, 1958.

Passmore R, Robson JS: A Companion to Medical Studies. Oxford: Blackwell, 1974.

Shepherd JA: A Concise Surgery of the Acute Abdomen. Edinburgh: Churchill, Livingstone, 1975.

Chapter 5

Physical Examination of the Abdomen

The aim of physical examination of the abdomen is to acquire as much evidence as possible in order to understand the location, extent, and nature of disease or lack of it. Examination must be thorough and must always include examination of the neck, chest, legs, back, groins, rectum, and female pelvis. Accurate examination is very informative but deceptively difficult. In this chapter only a few important points related to diagnosis of abdominal pain are described. No attempt is made to describe techniques of physical examination in detail since these are available in many excellent textbooks (2-5).

Accurate and complete physical examination of the abdomen is very important in the search for the cause of abdominal pain. Positive findings on physical examination must be considered strong evidence in contrast to vague symptoms or slightly abnormal laboratory results. A complete physical examination may reveal disease not associated with symptoms. When associated with appropriate history, some clinical findings on examination of the abdomen can lead directly to a working diagnosis (9). For example, if there is a history of midgut visceral pain, a gastrointestinal disturbance in the form of anorexia, nausea, or vomiting, and a point of maximum tenderness and muscle guarding in the right lower quadrant of the abdomen, the patient must be suspected of having acute appendicitis. In the gallbladder region tenderness, muscle guarding, and Murphy's sign are highly suggestive of acute cholecystitis. If one can feel the swollen, tender fundus of the gallbladder, the diagnosis is certain. The nontender, enlarged gallbladder in a patient who has jaundice and who has had recent weight loss is highly suggestive of malignant tumor obstruction of the lower common bile duct. The liver is usually enlarged and tender in acute hepatitis, and enlarged and firm but not tender in fatty infiltration. A firm, swollen, immobile, tender sigmoid colon strongly supports the diagnosis of acute diverticulitis, whereas the sigmoid colon is more mobile and less tender in the spastic colon. Crampy abdominal pain, vomiting, abdominal distension, obstipation, visible peristalsis, and hyperactive intestinal sounds are typical of bowel obstruction. As hypertension develops in the portal venous system, the liver may shrink, the spleen enlarge. There are many characteristic physical findings in patients having disease in the abdomen.

Physical examination of the abdomen should be performed under ideal conditions. The examining table should be firm, flat, and at a comfortable height for the examiner. The patient should be made comfortable and kept warm. There should be good lighting, preferably oblique and shining neither into the patient's nor the examiner's eyes. Examination of a patient in bed is not ideal. It is indiscreet to have a patient unduly exposed during examination. Physical examination of the abdomen must be considered incomplete if it is attempted under less than ideal conditions.

There is no excuse for roughness during examination. Much more accurate information is obtained from gentle palpation than from rough handling. An examination that causes unwarranted pain is likely to be inaccurate and incomplete because the patient becomes uncooperative. When a maneuver is painful, it should be kept brief and done accurately so that it will not have to be repeated. Rough maneuvers, such as shaking the pelvis or pounding on the lower ribs, are unnecessarily painful and rarely needed. The aim of physical examination of the abdomen is to gather as much evidence as possible deliberately and accurately.

Every examiner must learn a system for complete examination of the abdomen and related regions. A careful examiner will note unexpected findings that warrant eventual explanation. Guard against bias and avoid searching only for expected abnormalities. Correct interpretation of findings on physical examination of the abdomen is possible only if one is aware of the variations of normalcy. There may be an inferior extension of the lower border of the right lobe of the liver, a Riedel's lobe. Some patients, especially young adult females, are found to have solid stool filling the cecum, producing a right lower quadrant abdominal mass. In muscular and tense men the segments of the rectus abdominis muscle may be easily palpated and confused with an intra-abdominal mass. If the transverse and sigmoid parts of the colon are full, they may cause masses in thin patients. Lordosis causes the aorta and sometimes the pancreas to become prominent and palpable. If a female patient has a vaginal tampon in place, it is felt as a mass anteriorly on rectal examination. In the elderly an atrophic anterior abdominal wall may allow peristaltic movements of the intestine to be seen. Although examination of the abdomen and related regions is important in the assessment of abdominal pain, physical examination cannot be considered complete until all parts of the body are examined (Figure 12).

GENERAL APPEARANCES

During history taking the examiner will have noted the patient's apparent age and any obvious physical characteristics, and will have gained an impression of the patient's reactivity and degree of anxiety. The patient's facial expression reveals much. Does the patient appear seriously ill, debilitated, or excessively anxious? Patients who are chronically ill or toxemic often have a dull gaze and an ashen complexion. The patient who is bleeding or in shock appears pale and anxious and has cold perspiration on the brow. After prolonged

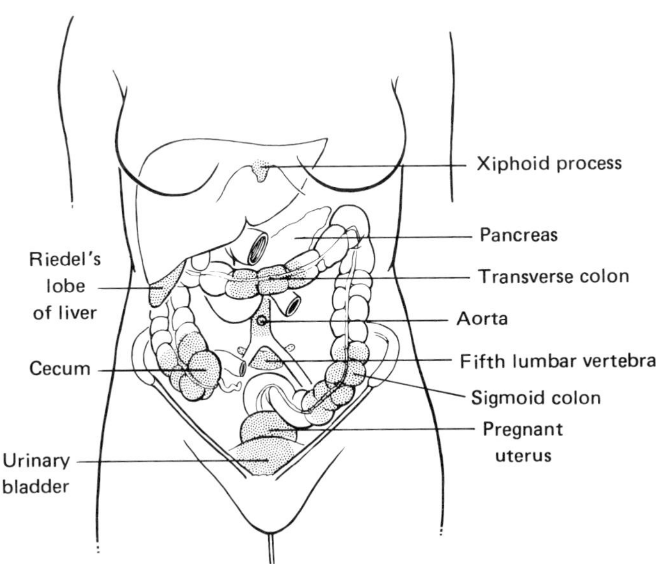

Figure 12 Masses that may be found on palpation of the normal abdomen. A tense rectus abdominis muscle may cause a palpable abdominal wall mass. Feces in the cecum or sigmoid parts of the colon, the rectus muscles, and a Riedel's lobe of the liver are the only normal masses off the midline.

vomiting and dehydration the cheeks and eyeballs appear sunken. Short, shallow, labored breathing may be associated with an overwhelming infection. Deathly pallor; gasping respirations; and pale lips, tongue, cheeks, and conjunctivas are characteristic in massive hemorrhage. Any serious illness may be associated with dehydration, confusion, and inappropriate behavior. An examiner should notice the odor associated with gastrointestinal hemorrhage, a fecal fistula, or ketosis. If the patient is black, remember the association of sickle cell trait with abdominal pain. If the patient with recurrent abdominal pain is from the Mediterranean basin, remember the possibility of episodic peritonitis with familial Mediterranean fever.

The physical attitude of the patient may be revealing. The patient with intestinal colic, biliary colic, renal colic, or a full bladder moves frequently. Injured patients might be restless because of confusion, severe hemorrhage, cerebral irritation, hypoxia, a full bladder, or an unsplinted fracture. On the other hand patients with peritonitis lie quietly on their backs, often with their hips and knees bent. With peritonitis or other painful lesion in the upper abdomen, the patient uses the upper thorax for breathing; there is little diaphragmatic or abdominal wall movement. Severe biliary colic or myocardial ischemic pain is often associated with splinting and immobility of the lower chest and upper abdomen. Patients with acute pancreatitis or pancreatic carcinoma may prefer to sit and lean forward supporting the abdomen with their arms or bent knees. Laborious breathing with active use of the accessory muscles of respiration and dilation of the nares is characteristic in pneumonia.

The pulse is likely to be more rapid in severe illness, but at the beginning of the illness it may be normal. Pulse irregularity may suggest a cardiac cause for abdominal pain, such as mesenteric embolus with intestinal infarction. A slow regular pulse generally indicates that there has been tolerance of the disease up to that time. Fever and a rapid pulse accompany inflammation. If there is no fever and the pulse is rapid and weakening, one should suspect hemorrhage or another cause for hypovolemia.

The body temperature should be considered in relation to the pulse rate. (In ill patients the temperature is best taken rectally.) High temperatures are quite unusual in the early stages of surgical abdominal disease (1). A mild fever may be associated with bleeding or a malignancy. Most often a fever indicates infection and inflammation. The highest fevers tend to be associated with pneumonia or kidney infections. High fever, falling blood pressure, and rapid pulse mean septic shock; infection in a closed space must be sought and drained. Patients in shock or severely debilitated may have subnormal body temperature. If fever is expected yet absent in patients having severe infection, it must be assumed that the patient's ability to respond to stress is poor.

INSPECTION

Inspection of the abdomen is best carried out with the patient comfortably supine with one or two pillows under the head, arms at the sides, and the legs straight or the knees drawn up. For inspection of the abdomen the trunk should be exposed from the nipples to the pubis. It is important to have the urinary bladder empty before rectal and pelvic examinations otherwise pelvic masses may be missed. The size and contour of the abdomen are noted. Is the patient generally obese or is there the appearance of abdominal enlargement? General inspection may reveal the presence of a mass. In general, abdominal wall veins are not prominent. If veins are prominent, the direction of flow in these veins should be determined. It would be abnormal if the flow in enlarged abdominal wall veins were away from the umbilicus, upward from the groins to the axilla, or downward from the axilla to the groins. Portal hypertension, obstruction of the inferior vena cava or obstruction of the superior vena cava could be the abnormality in each case.

Careful note of the respiratory movements should be made. As a rule respiratory movements are mainly abdominal in diseases of the chest and mainly upper thoracic in painful diseases of the upper abdomen and lower chest. Breathing tends to be shallow in peritonitis to reduce painful movement of the diaphragm and abdominal wall. Gasping respirations are characteristic with hemorrhage or extensive chest disease. Is the respiratory movement of the abdominal wall greater on one side? If so, it might indicate restriction on the opposite side because of nearby inflammation, such as acute cholecystitis. This effect may be more obvious if the patient is asked to take a deep breath. A deep breath may cause shoulder top pain caused by stimulation of the central portion of the diaphragm. Respiratory movements make the pain of pleurisy worse. The site of an inflammation may be revealed if the patient is asked to draw the abdomen inward. Similarly the patient may be able to indicate the site of pain by bloating the abdomen outward or by coughing or sneezing.

The anterior abdominal wall should be observed both from the foot and from the side of the bed. The examiner's eyes should be at the level of the anterior abdominal wall to properly examine for swelling. One should look for a mass that might be an enlarged organ, a hernia, or an abnormal mass caused by disease. Intestinal peristalsis may be seen in the elderly if the abdominal wall is thin and relaxed. In the newborn with hypertrophic pyloric stenosis left to right peristaltic waves may be seen in the distended epigastrium prior to vomiting. In distal colonic obstruction peristaltic waves in the transverse colon might be observed to pass from right to left. Small bowel peristaltic movements are observed in the middle of the abdomen and move in any direction.

The umbilicus is deep in the obese. Because of poor hygiene, inflammation may occur in a deep umbilicus, causing reddening at the edges and a discharge. Paraumbilical hernia is common in obese adults.

PALPATION

Abdominal muscle reflexes are tested by lightly stroking the skin in each of the four abdominal quadrants; this testing should be carried out prior to palpation. At this time one can test also for anesthesia, hyperalgesia, and hyperesthesia. Palpation of the abdomen is more informative if performed before administration of narcotics that relax and relieve pain. The examiner's hands should be warm. Gentleness is much better than roughness. Palpation at first should be light; followed by deeper palpation in the absence of tenderness.

Palpation is begun in the quadrant where it is believed there is least tenderness. In turn other quadrants are examined. Gentle indentation of the abdominal wall is used to test for the tenseness of the abdominal wall muscles. There is every variation between voluntary muscle guarding of the abdominal wall muscles in an anxious or excited individual to a very tight abdominal wall found in the typical boardlike rigidity of a patient with a perforated duodenal ulcer. Gentle palpation is used in all parts of the abdomen for areas of tenderness, masses, or enlarged organs.

A MASS

Nothing appears to excite a general surgeon more than an abdominal mass. If abnormal, it is objective evidence that disease is present. Diagnosis is often possible from the characteristics of the mass on clinical examination alone. A physician may consider the examination of an abdominal mass a sport, for the odds may be against getting the correct answer. Students are expected to make the correct diagnosis every time (8).

The diagnostic possibilities of an abdominal mass include an enlarged normal organ; a normal organ out of place; an organ distended with secretion; or a congenital, traumatic, inflammatory, vascular, neoplastic, or degenerative lesion. In spite of the many possibilities, the probability of making a correct diagnosis is increased by a systematic examination of the characteristics of the mass, as follows:

Site	Motility
Size	Tenderness
Shape	Overlying skin
Edges	Discharge
Surface	Sinus
Consistency	Fistula
Mobility	

The site of an abdominal mass may suggest its cause. The examiner should consider normal structures at that site, although some organs may wander. The size of the mass should be noted and if possible measurements should be taken in three dimensions. Where it is impossible to measure, an estimate is made. The shape of a mass may suggest that it is a normal resident of that region of the abdomen. Cysts are spherical or ovoid. The edges of a mass may be well defined and discrete or poorly defined. The edges of a hernia are discrete, whereas the edges of an inflammatory mass or an infiltrating tumor are obscure. The surface of the mass may be smooth or irregular and uneven. It may be lobulated as if it were made up of many elements. Nodularity suggests spherical masses arising from the surface of the main mass. A craggy surface suggests irregular hardness with projections and is the term applied to the surface characteristics of some malignant neoplasms.

The consistency of a mass may be difficult to describe, varying from soft fluidity to rock hardness. Compressibility suggests that the mass decreases in size with pressure as does a hernia or hemangioma. Elasticity means compressibility with instantaneous return to its former size. Fluctuation implies compressibility in all directions so that there is transmitted elasticity. Percussion may distinguish gas from fluid, and transillumination may distinguish fluid from solid. The mobility of a mass depends upon adjacent structures. The motility of a mass refers to its intrinsic movement. There may be a transmitted pulse, a peristaltic movement, or an expansion on coughing. The tenderness of a mass is always determined. The skin overlying the mass may show discoloration, fixation, edema, or inflammation, or may undergo ulceration.

Discharge related to a mass may arise from the surface, a sinus, or a fistula. Sinuses result from retained foreign bodies such as drains, gauze, bullets or other missiles, necrotic soft tissues, necrotic bone or cartilage, chronic or specific infections such as tuberculosis or actinomycosis, or from the rigidity of the walls of cavities that prevent collapse and closure. A fistula may persist because of a distal obstruction, reinfection, epithelial lining, foreign body, or neoplasm. Both sinuses and fistulas heal slowly if the region is ischemic or has been irradiated, if the patient is in poor general condition, or if the patient has received adrenocorticosteroid or immunosuppressive therapy.

Palpation is used to check abdominal organs for enlargement and the reason for enlargement. There may be general enlargement or focal enlargement with nodularity. Careful examination of the usual sites of hernia is important for diagnosis of the cause of abdominal pain. There may be a mass produced by an irreducible hernia or there may be nothing more than tenderness at the exact site of a hernial orifice. The inguinal canal, the femoral canal, the umbilicus, and the epigastric midline should be examined for hernias.

The exact location of tenderness is important. Point tenderness in the usual site of the appendix may be the most significant finding in early appendicitis. The point of tenderness in kidney disease is the angle between the twelfth rib and the lateral border of sacrospinalis muscle. Tenderness in the epigastrium is the only physical finding in uncomplicated duodenal ulcer disease. Percussion may be used to confirm palpation. For example, suspected minor liver enlargement may be more accurately assessed by percussion. The extent of the area of tympany on percussion of the gastric air bubble may be used to rule out splenic enlargement. Tenderness may be confined to the abdominal wall (10).

Palpation is a very important part of the assessment of disease of the abdomen. Examination of the site of tenderness, the tenseness of the overlying abdominal muscles, and the finding of an enlarged organ or a mass can be most rewarding. Examination of the abdomen should be repeated often to fully assess the pain problem. Although it is essential to document the examination beforehand, it may be revealing to reexamine the abdomen after sedation, analgesics, or anesthesia. In these cases deeper palpation is easier because pain is relieved and muscles are relaxed, and previously hidden masses may be found.

Different types of tenderness may be associated with peritonitis. They include local tenderness, remote tenderness, local rebound tenderness, and remote rebound tenderness. Local tenderness or tenderness on direct pressure is always found over an inflammation. Remote tenderness refers to pain that is produced at the site of inflammation with pressure on some remote part of the abdomen. The palm of the hand may be used to apply steady pressure over an area on the opposite side of the abdomen. In appendicitis, pain produced at McBurney's point with pressure on the left lower quadrant is called Rovsing's sign. Local rebound tenderness refers to pain produced at the site of an inflammation with abrupt release from pressure directly over this site. Sometimes this is better produced by repeated light tapping than by sudden release of a single press. Remote rebound tenderness refers to pain produced at the site of inflammation with sudden release of pressure from some remote part of the abdomen. This is considered a sign of peritoneal irritation, but it is not as important as guarding of the muscles overlying an inflammation.

Pay special attention to the femoral and inguinal orifices and make certain there is no mass or tenderness. Note whether both testicles have descended. Check the femoral pulses, an absent pulse may be the clue for a dissecting aneurysm or acute occlusion of the abdominal aorta. Always examine for lymph node enlargements in the neck, axillas, and groins.

PERCUSSION

Percussion may cause the patient undue distress. It is wise to begin percussion where it is least likely to be painful. Percussion is used as a check on palpation to evaluate the sizes of organs, such as the liver and the spleen. Percussion may be used as a method of comparing tenderness from quadrant to quadrant. Single finger percussion may be used to confirm local tenderness provided it is performed gently. Percussion may be used to map out areas of abdominal tenderness. The percussion note over abnormal abdominal masses may be important. Dullness indicates a solid or fluid-filled mass, whereas tympany indicates gas. Percussion is commonly used on abdominal examination to diagnose a distended urinary bladder. In the flank dullness to percussion is expected. Shifting dullness means that free fluid is present in the peritoneal cavity. There is nonshifting dullness over a hematoma, around a bleeding tubal pregnancy, or around a ruptured spleen. In other areas of the abdomen in such cases the fluid is nonclotting and shifting dullness is found.

Closed fist percussion of the right lower chest wall to demonstrate liver or gallbladder tenderness is painful and rarely needed. Gentle palpation on deep inspiration is more accurate and less painful.

AUSCULTATION

Physicians must be familiar with normal intestinal sounds, which are heard at least once every 2 minutes. Bowel sounds can occur only when fluid and air are present together in the intestine. If no gas is present in the bowel, no bowel sounds are heard. Intestinal sounds become abnormal when they are greatly decreased or greatly increased in loudness and frequency. Absence of intestinal sounds means absence of air in the intestine or absence of organized peristaltic activity. Absence of intestinal sounds for a period of 2 minutes *usually* means paralytic ileus, which is always secondary and has many causes (Chapter 8). Paralytic ileus occurs under anesthesia and in the early postoperative period when peristaltic waves are disorganized. After a period of 30–48 hours following laparotomy, peristaltic sounds return and soon afterward gas is passed by rectum. These signs indicate the return of organized peristalsis, and oral feedings may be resumed with safety. A complete truncal vagotomy doubles the duration of postlaparotomy paralytic ileus.

An increase in loudness and frequency of intestinal sounds means increased peristaltic activity, as in acute gastroenteritis. In mechanical obstruction of the bowel there are repeated cyclic waves that coincide with the cramps. The bowel sounds are loud and hyperactive, increasing in crescendo fashion to a final loud noise, and then rapidly decreasing to a few tinkles between cramps.

Some patients are so frightened of tenderness that they will not allow abdominal palpation. One trick that can be tried is to palpate while holding a stethoscope chest piece in the examining hand; patients do not associate the pressure of a stethoscope with pain on palpation.

Auscultation may occasionally reveal a friction rub over the liver or spleen. It is sometimes difficult to rule out a nearby pleural or pericardial friction rub. A pericardial friction rub does not stop if the breath is held. A friction rub results from two rough surfaces moving against one another; the rub disappears if fluid separates the rough surfaces.

Auscultation may reveal a bruit over a major vessel that might indicate eddying at irregularities or narrowings. This observation may be of diagnostic importance when found just above and lateral to the umbilicus, over the renal arteries. A bruit over the celiac artery may be found in normal individuals (7). Occasionally a venous hum can be heard over dilated umbilical veins at the umbilicus when the portal venous pressure is high.

A succussion splash may be heard with or without a stethoscope. It is almost always an indication of a large amount of both fluid and air in an enlarged stomach. A succussion splash is normally found in a newborn or infant who has been fed but not burped. It is often found in young adults who have drunk a large amount of ale. If a succussion splash is detected 3 hours after a meal it means delayed emptying or pyloric narrowing or occlusion. Succussion splashes are initiated by body movement, either gentle shaking or repeated percussion of the abdominal wall with the patient suitably relaxed in a semisitting position. Borborygmi are exaggerated peristaltic sounds heard without a stethoscope; they are independent of body movement.

The upper third of the peritoneal cavity lies deep to the lower ribs and is not accessible to clinical examination except by percussion. For this reason subphrenic abscess is often difficult to diagnose, and tumors in the upper half of the stomach are rarely palpable. At least one-fourth of the peritoneal cavity lies within the pelvis. Abdominal, rectal, and pelvic examinations are essential components of the clinical examination of the lower abdomen and pelvis.

Beware of overlooking serious disease in the aged and in infants. At the extremes of life patients show less reaction to disease than at other ages. Immunosuppressive drugs and adrenocortical steroid hormones alter the normal responses of the body to stress and repair and therefore the responses to infection and wound healing are altered. Serious infection may develop with few if any signs of illness, and healing may be greatly delayed.

RECTAL AND PELVIC EXAMINATION

Examination of the abdomen is considered incomplete until a rectal examination is performed. Unless there is painful disease of the anal canal rectal examination should never be deferred. In the female further information can be obtained from bimanual pelvic examination. These examinations are more accurate if the bowel and bladder are empty.

ANCILLARY EXAMINATIONS

Ancillary examinations are most important in the search for some causes of abdominal pain. Esophagoscopy is important for diagnosis of esophageal strictures, neoplasms, ulcers, and esophagitis. Gastroscopy reveals peptic ulcer, gastric neoplasms, and other gastric and duodenal lesions. Speculum examination of the cervix and anoscopic and sigmoidoscopic examinations of the anal canal and rectum may reveal the cause of pelvic pain; these examinations are simple and should be part of a complete physical examination. With experience peritoneoscopy or laparoscopy may be helpful in examining the liver, abdominal masses, and the female pelvic organs. The characteristics and relationships of a mass or cyst can be further defined by ultrasonography and computerized axial tomography in addition to other radiological and isotopic examinations.

In recording the physical examination concentrate on describing the observation rather than interpreting what has been found. The ideal time for objective review of all of the evidence is at the conclusion of the physical examination. If evidence is analyzed at that time, it will not be impaired by previous interpretations and judgments.

ACCURACY IN CLINICAL EXAMINATION

Accuracy in clinical examination comes from consistency and uniformity. Where standard techniques are used, the appreciation of physical abnormalities is more accurate and reliable. Do not hesitate to have an experienced colleague examine the patient for confirmation of physical findings. Accuracy of clinical examination and diagnosis is established through feedback by diagnostic laboratory investigations including X-rays, exposure of the disease at surgery, response to specific treatment, and postmortem examination.

Physical examination of the abdomen can be very rewarding in the diagnosis of abdominal pain. It appears to be easy but it is not. With care and experience the examination can become remarkably accurate and informative. Omission of careful examination of the abdomen and rectum may be tragic for the patient and disgraceful for the physician.

REFERENCES

1. Cope Z: The Early Diagnosis of the Acute Abdomen, 14th ed. London: Oxford, 1972.
2. DeGowin EL, DeGowin RL: Bedside Diagnostic Examination, 3d ed. New York: MacMillan, 1976.
3. Delp MH, Manning RT: Major's Physical Diagnosis, 8th ed. Philadelphia: Saunders, 1975.
4. Judge RD, Zuidema GD: Methods of Clinical Examination. Boston: Little, Brown, 1974.
5. Kampmeier RH, Blake TM: Physical Examination in Health and Disease, 4th ed. Philadelphia: Davis, 1970.

6. Kingsnorth AN: Fluid filled intestinal obstruction. Br J Surg 63:289–291, 1976.
7. Marston A, Kieny R, Szilagyi E, Taylor GW: Intestinal ischemia. Arch Surg 111:107–112, 1976.
8. Perkins G: The Foundations of Surgery. Edinburgh: Livingstone, 1954.
9. Smith JN: Essentials of Gastroenterology. St. Louis: Mosby, 1969.
10. Thomson H, Francis DMA: Abdominal-wall tenderness; a useful sign in the acute abdomen. Lancet 2:1053–1054, 1977.

Chapter 6

Laboratory Investigation

A discussion of all laboratory aids that might be useful in the investigation of a patient with abdominal pain could easily fill a large textbook. It would be unreasonable to attempt even a summary of all such investigations in this chapter. Investigations that could be considered diagnostic are in Chapters 7 and 8. This chapter reviews laboratory aids to diagnosis of acute abdominal conditions with general remarks on elective laboratory investigations for less urgent cases.

EMERGENCY LABORATORY INVESTIGATION

Sudden onset of severe abdominal pain is an indication for rapid diagnosis. Often such cases are serious and need early surgical treatment. Delay may reduce the chance of survival. Early diagnosis is based partly on a few simple laboratory investigations. These investigations should be kept to a minimum and should be performed and interpreted without delay. The following are the most useful.

White Blood Cell Count

A white blood cell (leukocyte) count is a useful and practical aid. Serial counts are more reliable than single counts; however, the leukocyte count is subject to ±10% error. Never change a diagnosis on the basis of a 20% difference between two counts.

The white blood cell count is often normal in the earliest stages of sudden onset diseases. In infants, the aged, the malnourished, and the chronically ill the responses of the body are less predictable and the blood cell counts may remain normal longer than in other patients. A normal leukocyte count does not rule out an active infection.

In the initial assessment of patients with acute abdominal pain, an elevated leukocyte count usually means there is an active infection or inflammatory process somewhere in the body. Occasionally it may be the first evidence of an inflammation. As a rule the white blood cell count provides supporting evidence for diagnosis of an inflammatory disease, such as acute appendicitis; however, a normal leukocyte count must not dissuade a physician from a clinical diagnosis. In acute appendicitis or inflammation in other hollow organs, rapidly rising or unusually high leukocyte counts may portend empyema, gangrene, or perforation. Very high leukocyte counts are frequently associated with diseases outside the gastrointestinal tract, such as pneumonia, pyelonephritis, or pelvic inflammatory disease.

A raised leukocyte count may be found in acute abdominal conditions unrelated to bacterial infection. Such conditions include perforation of a duodenal ulcer, hemorrhage or torsion of an ovarian cyst, abdominal trauma, and intraperitoneal hemorrhage.

Serious infection need not be associated with elevated leukocyte counts. Gram-negative septicemia and acute typhoid enterocolitis are examples in which stippled leukocytes may be found. Leukopenia may be the result of an overwhelming infection. Some inflammatory diseases, especially those believed to be caused by viruses, are usually not accompanied by a raised leukocyte count. Such diseases include mesenteric lymphadenitis and common acute gastroenteritis. A patient may have an undiagnosed blood disease with an altered leukocyte count before developing an abdominal complication or an unrelated abdominal condition. For instance, leukopenia, leukemia, or mononucleosis may have been present before the abdominal crisis. Thus, it is important to know what cells make up the white blood cell count.

Examination of the Blood Smear

An increase in numbers of polymorphonuclear leukocytes, especially young neutrophils, usually indicates a bacterial infection. In viral infections there is often a relative lymphocytosis. A lymphocytosis or monocytosis may be seen in malaria or tuberculosis. Lymphocytosis may also occur in acute adrenocortical insufficiency. Eosinophilia is often found in hypersensitivity reactions and parasitic infestations.

Examination of a thick blood film may reveal the malaria organism. Malaria is still endemic in parts of Central and South America, Africa, and Asia. Because malaria can mimic many diseases, it should be considered in all ill travelers from these regions.

Sickle-cell disease is caused by inherited abnormal hemoglobin that crystallizes with anoxia. Allowing a wet smear of red blood cells to stand for a time under a cover slip sealed with petroleum jelly results in sickling. Patients with sickle-cell disease may have abdominal pain caused by multiple microinfarcts in any organ including the spleen. Patients of black ancestry who are anemic and have abdominal pain should be suspected of having sickle-cell disease.

Hematocrit

The hematocrit is a measure of the packed cell volume expressed as a percentage of the whole blood volume. Since red blood cells far outnumber other blood cells, the hematocrit is almost equivalent to the hemoglobin; both indicate hemoglobin concentration.

In acute hemorrhage, plasma and cells are lost in normal proportions; so the hematocrit and hemoglobin are misleadingly normal at first. As extravascular fluid enters the blood stream, hemodilution occurs. This effect is enhanced by administration of electrolyte solutions that make the hematocrit fall more rapidly. Remember this change when attempting to estimate blood loss by the hematocrit; at best it is a very rough guide. Preexisting anemia may confuse the picture. Adequacy of blood volume replacement is indicated most reliably by a number of parameters in addition to the hematocrit, such as vital signs, central venous pressure, hourly urine output, and the general condition of the patient.

A patient who has been vomiting becomes dehydrated, and the degree of dehydration is reflected in the hematocrit. As parenteral fluids are given, the hematocrit falls toward normal (2).

Urinalysis

Urinalysis is simple but important. Urine should always be tested as part of the initial examination. The color of normal urine suggests its specific gravity. Accurate measurement of specific gravity is a simple, practical substitute for urine osmolality in the emergency room. Hemoconcentration should be associated with concentrated urine, and hemodilution with dilute urine. Hypovolemia, shock, and reduced renal perfusion are associated with low volume and increased concentration of urine, if renal function is otherwise normal. Dilute urine in the face of hemoconcentration suggests renal disease.

Renal infection or disease may be discovered by pyuria, hematuria, albuminuria, or renal casts in the urine. Uncontrolled diabetics, especially young diabetics in ketoacidosis, often have a bizarre type of abdominal pain, and the main clue is sugar detected on urinalysis. A urine sample that is dark or turns dark may be the first sign of porphyria, a metabolic cause for abdominal pain.

Serum Amylase

Serum amylase is most helpful in diagnosis of acute pancreatitis. It must be performed in all problematic cases of acute abdominal pain. A slight elevation of serum amylase is not diagnostic of acute pancreatitis, although this may occur early in the disease or with almost complete necrosis of the pancreas. The serum amylase becomes diagnostic only when it reaches a value five times the upper limit of normal. Amylase is excreted in the urine, and therefore impaired renal function may cause an elevation of the serum amylase in the absence of pancreatic disease. The urine amylase concentration remains elevated longer than the serum amylase concentration and is therefore more helpful than the serum amylase in detecting transient attacks of pancreatitis and in making the diagnosis later in the disease.

Other Less Immediate Laboratory Tests

Other tests may be performed when indicated. Diarrhea stools may be examined for pus, parasites, or blood. Discharge from the vagina, urethra, fistulas, or draining wounds should be sampled for microscopic examination and bacterial culture.

Any fluid obtained by paracentesis, peritoneal lavage, or thoracentesis should be examined for bacteria, leukocytes, erythrocytes, and amylase concentration. Special examinations such as sigmoidoscopy, gastroscopy, and bronchoscopy may be needed to evaluate injuries or disease, to obtain bacteriological or pathological specimens, or to carry out treatments such as decompression of a sigmoid volvulus.

For preoperative assessment tests that may be ordered include blood urea nitrogen, serum creatinine, fasting blood sugar, serum electrolytes, blood gases, and electrocardiogram.

Ultrasonography has proven to be valuable in the rapid assessment of patients with abdominal pain where examination for masses, fluid collections, or calculi are indicated. Ultrasonography is useful in the investigation of gallbladder disease, extrahepatic obstructive jaundice, liver abscess, pancreatic cyst or mass, aortic aneurysm, splenic hematoma, and renal and perirenal masses. Also it may be helpful in the search for an intraperitoneal abscess, especially in the subphrenic, pelvic, and retroperitoneal parts of the abdomen.

EMERGENCY RADIOLOGICAL EXAMINATIONS

Most patients with acute abdominal disease have plain X-rays of the abdomen and chest despite the fact that the diagnosis may be clinically apparent. Because of the hour the primary care physician may have to interpret films without expert help. A radiologist, if available, needs adequate clinical information. Always be sure that the quality of the films is satisfactory and that the entire abdomen and chest are shown. The patient should be encouraged to void before plain film examination. If there is any suspicion of retention, catheterization should be carried out. The usual films are erect, supine, and left lateral decubitus views of the abdomen and posteroanterior and lateral views of the chest. Ill patients may not tolerate the erect position so that supine and left lateral decubitus views of the abdomen as well as a supine view of the chest may be all that can be obtained.

One method for systematic examination of an X-ray film consists of examining: (a) all of the bones and joints; (b) the soft tissues, normal viscera, abdominal wall, and any abnormal shadows; (c) gas shadows, normal or abnormal, within the intestinal tract, peritoneal cavity, or elsewhere; (d) opacities such as calcification in normal structures or abnormal calcifications; (e) general view of the whole film from a distance (5). Never stop after recognizing an obvious abnormality; always examine the entire film.

When viewing films of patients with abdominal pain, one might see a fresh fracture that suggests that the abdominal pain is a complication of a recent injury. Osteoporosis, metastasis, or a collapsed vertebra might be the cause of the pain. In examining the soft tissues it should be remembered that the extraperitoneal fatty layer in the flanks disappears with the edema of a nearby infection. The lateral border of the psoas muscle may not be seen because of inflammatory edema or retroperitoneal hemorrhage. However, absence of a psoas shadow in a perfectly well patient is not uncommon. Gas and fat are less dense than water by X-ray. Water-dense organs such as the liver, spleen, kidneys, and urinary bladder are observable. They are usually outlined by fat. Shadows that are more dense than water include the bones, calcifications in organs, and some foreign bodies. An abnormal soft tissue shadow might be an aneurysm, neoplasm, or abscess.

Gas in the bowel usually shows the mucosa in characteristic patterns. In health very little gas is seen in the small bowel by X-ray except in young children. Gas is normally present in the colon and stomach. The rugal folds of the stomach are usually evident in the left upper quadrant. The colon is distinguished by haustral folds, fecal material, and its peripheral location. In the peritoneal cavity gas shows up best on an erect or left lateral decubitus film. In the left lateral decubitus film the right side of the patient is uppermost and there is no gastric air bubble in the right upper quadrant to create confusion. These films, if properly made, can show 1-2 milliliters of air from a ruptured hollow viscus. On a supine film there must be a large quantity of intraperitoneal gas to be recognized. Intraperitoneal gas outlines the serosa of the bowel, whereas intraluminal gas is outlined by the mucosal surface. Occasionally gas can be identified within the wall of the bowel, which indicates gangrene. Often a subdiaphragmatic air-fluid level is seen best on an erect film of the chest. Gas in the gallbladder or bile ducts might accompany gallstone ileus with cholecystduodenal fistula, or follow choledochoduodenostomy or sphincteroplasty. In the intrahepatic portal venous branches gas is usually a premorbid development in intestinal strangulation and gangrene in adults. Gas may be seen in the wall of the gallbladder in emphysematous cholecystitis and in the wall of the urinary bladder in emphysematous cystitis.

Examples in films of greater-than-water-density shadows that can be encountered in an acute abdominal condition are gallstones, urinary tract calculi, appendiceal fecaliths, calcified abdominal aneurysms, pancreatic calcifications, and small bowel gallstones. Calcified lymph nodes, phleboliths in the pelvis, calcified uterine fibroids, and calcifications in small vessels are often seen on plain films and are seldom significant.

Chest films may show an intrathoracic cause for abdominal pain such as pneumonia. Chest X-rays occasionally demonstrate findings more directly related to the abdominal disease such as pulmonary metastasis, esophageal hiatus hernia, or rupture of the diaphragm. Pleural effusion either with atelectasis or without apparent pulmonary disease should suggest inflammation nearby in the abdomen, especially subphrenic abscess or acute pancreatitis, the former more commonly on the right side, the latter on the left.

Intestinal obstruction is associated with air-fluid levels and gaseous distension proximal to the occlusion. It is important to know whether the patient has had a sigmoidoscopic or colonoscopic examination or a cleansing enema prior to the examination since these can introduce gas into the colon and lead to false interpretation. Air-fluid levels are seen on either an erect or lateral decubitus view of the abdomen; a supine view shows wide loops of gas-filled bowel. Air is normally seen in the stomach and colon. The colon must be dilated or have long air-fluid levels to suggest obstruction. Remember that the differentiation of bowel obstruction and paralytic ileus rests primarily on history and clinical examination. The essential features of various gas patterns are summarized in Table 4 (3).

Gas-filled loops of bowel may be separated by edema or hemorrhage in the bowel wall or may be separated by intraperitoneal free fluid as a result of a transudate, exudate, perforation, or hemorrhage. Localized paralytic ileus may produce a single loop of bowel filled with gas or gas and fluid causing an air-fluid level. This may lie beside an inflamed organ, a sentinel loop. A closed

Table 4 Gas Patterns on Plain Films of the Abdomen[a]

Primary observation	Discriminator	Possible diagnoses
No gas	No fluid	Protracted vomiting
	Fluid-filled loops	Closed loop obstruction Strangulated bowel Mesenteric vascular occlusion
Air–fluid levels and severe small bowel distension	No colonic air–fluid levels	Small bowel mechanical obstruction or paralytic ileus
	Air–fluid levels in the right colon	Right colonic obstruction Acute appendicitis Strangulated bowel Mesenteric vascular occlusion
Colonic distension with air–fluid levels	Without air in the rectum	Early colon obstruction Paralytic ileus
	With air in the rectum	Paralytic ileus Anal obstruction
Air–fluid levels in small bowel and colon and no gas in the rectum	Moderately dilated cecum	Mechanical obstruction Paralytic ileus (either, with incompetent ileocecal valve)
	Severely dilated cecum	Advanced colonic obstruction with competent ileocecal valve

[a]Adapted from Fisher, M. S., M.D.: The Analysis of Survey Abdominal Radiographs in Intestinal Ileus. Radiologic Science Update Series, W. J. Tuddenham, M.D., Editor, *1* #6, 1976, with permission of the author and editor.

loop obstruction may be outlined by an air–fluid level; probably more commonly, the involved segment of bowel is fluid filled and is presented radiographically as a tumorlike mass of water density. This false tumor sign must be differentiated clinically from the fluid filled loop of simple obstruction. Tenderness in the region of an abdominal mass that is apparent on X-ray must suggest the possibility of a strangulated loop of bowel. Thus, absence of air in part of the abdomen is an important sign in a patient with intestinal obstruction, especially if it is associated with a mass or tenderness in that region.

Intraperitoneal complications in the early postoperative period are difficult to diagnose. Free air remains in the peritoneal cavity for 1–8 days following laparotomy and is probably only related to the volume of air originally trapped. Obese patients tend to have less air trapped. It should be remembered that abdominal drains can rarely increase the quantity of air in the peritoneal cavity in the postoperative period. Anesthesia and surgical operation are associated with paralytic ileus, the duration of which doubles if truncal vagotomy is performed.

SPECIAL RADIOLOGICAL PROCEDURES FOR EMERGENCY CASES

Several radiological procedures involving the use of contrast media may be useful in the urgent investigation of patients with abdominal pain. Some thoughtful consideration should be given to the order of contrast studies. If there is any likelihood that an intravenous pyelogram, intravenous cholangiogram, or emergency arteriogram might be necessary, these procedures should be given priority over barium studies. If barium is introduced first, it must be cleared from the intestinal tract before other X-rays are taken.

Intravenous Pyelogram

An intravenous pyelogram shows the kidney in the nephrogram phase and the renal pelvis, ureters, and bladder in the excretory phase. It is the most useful contrast X-ray of the upper urinary tract, and the method of choice in establishing the diagnosis of urinary tract calculi. It can, if necessary, be done during laparotomy. In trauma it is valuable in showing damage on the side of injury and also the presence of a functioning kidney on the other side in case a decision must be made regarding removal of the injured organ. It is a function study of the upper urinary tract as opposed to the retrograde pyelogram. After severe trauma a kidney shown by intravenous pyelography to be nonfunctioning is not necessarily seriously damaged. Renal arteriography is necessary for further evaluation. Retrograde pyelograms are seldom indicated in the evaluation of patients with renal trauma.

Intravenous Cholangiography

Intravenous cholangiography is useful in emergency cases to diagnose acute cholecystitis and in such cases to reduce the likelihood of common duct exploration if cholecystectomy is to be performed. If the common bile duct is identified by intravenous cholangiography and the gallbladder fails to visualize over six hours, a diagnosis of cystic duct obstruction or acute cholecystitis can be made.

Barium Enema

A barium enema confirms colonic or rectal obstruction and often demonstrates its nature. It is contraindicated to give any enema, including a barium enema, to a patient with possible colonic perforation or peritoneal irritation. During exacerbations of ulcerative colitis or Crohn's disease, barium enema may precipitate toxic megacolon and should be avoided.

If the level of the occlusion of a bowel obstruction is not clear clinically, barium enema should be performed first, and then if the occlusion is not demonstrated, oral barium can be administered. Barium by mouth can locate obstructing lesions in the small intestine but should be not given until colonic obstruction has been excluded.

Gastrografin Swallow

Gastrografin swallow is occasionally used to demonstrate an atypical spontaneous rupture of the esophagus. It should not be needed for gastric or duodenal perforations.

Angiography

Angiography may be helpful in selected cases. Aortography is rarely needed or advised for palpable abdominal aneurysms, but it is often helpful for acute dissecting aneurysms. Abdominal angiography may be useful in investigating active gastrointestinal bleeding; rupture of solid organs such as liver, spleen, or kidney; and occasionally possible mesenteric arterial occlusion as causes of abdominal pain. The value of this procedure for these purposes is limited. Gastrointestinal bleeding must exceed 0.5 milliliter per minute in order to be demonstrable by arteriography.

Computed Body Tomography

Computed body tomography, with its unique thin section display of anatomic detail during life, is still in its infancy. With a modern scanner the scan time is within the breath-holding capacity of the patient, and much of the peristaltic activity and motion artifact is eliminated. Computed tomography is much more sensitive in detecting differences in tissue density than is conventional radiography. This factor, together with its noninvasive nature, makes computed tomography an extremely valuable tool in examination of the abdomen. Although its initial impact has not been as great in examination of the body as in the head, it has already established itself as the most useful diagnostic procedure in the retroperitoneal area. Its use will undoubtedly grow as we become more familiar with the appearance of the normal and various pathologic processes in the abdomen.

LABORATORY INVESTIGATION OF ELECTIVE CASES

As mentioned at the beginning of this chapter a complete survey of all possible laboratory investigations is outside the scope and intention of this book. However, a few remarks regarding the use of laboratory investigations will be made, emphasizing the need to be selective and to use investigations that have reasonable sensitivity, specificity, and accuracy.

Many of the more common laboratory tests must be considered an integral part of the clinical examination. Laboratory tests provide feedback to enhance the accuracy of the diagnosis made from history and physical examination. Some laboratory tests are highly specific and very sensitive and therefore can be considered diagnostic; some extend physical examination of the patient beyond the clinician's power, such as X-ray examinations and the concentration of respiratory gases in arterial blood; some detect asymptomatic or subclinical disease. This is the main argument for routine urinalysis, chest X-rays, electrocardiograms, blood cell counts, and blood smears. During treatment, laboratory tests may be used to monitor the concentrations and effects of drugs in the blood stream. Tests may demonstrate the response to treatment and the approach of recovery.

Physicians should be highly selective in ordering laboratory tests. There is no substitute for a complete and methodical clinical examination; the cost to the physician in time and effort is amply repaid by personal satisfaction and the patient's gratitude. Excessive laboratory test results tax the physician's power of analysis and some positive results may be overlooked. Selective use of laboratory investigations prevents the frustration and inaccuracy of an overburdened laboratory and helps control medical costs. Physicians should not underrate clinical evidence. Where accurate history and accurate physical examination make the diagnosis, laboratory tests are not only unnecessary but wasteful.

As a rule immediate evidence that is personally seen, felt, or heard is more reliable than mediate evidence received verbally or in a written report; the mediator must be considered an additional possible source of error (8).

A perceptive tongue-in-cheek list of reasons why physicians order laboratory tests has been written by Asher (1):

> 1 I order this test because, if it agrees with my opinion I will believe it, and if it does not I shall disbelieve it.
>
> 2 I do not understand this test and am uncertain of the normal figure, but it is the fashion to order it.
>
> 3 When my Chief asks if you have done this or that test I like to say, yes, so I order as many tests as I can to avoid being caught out.
>
> 4 I have no clear idea of what I am looking for, but in ordering this test I feel in a vague way that something might turn up.
>
> 5 I order this test because I want to convince the patient that there is nothing wrong and I don't think he will believe me without a test. (p. 167)

To this list one might add: "I order this test because some day in court a lawyer might ask me if I did this test, and if not, why not?"

ANALYSIS OF TEST RESULTS FROM THE LABORATORY

Results from laboratory tests are expressed in one of two ways, either as a number or as a classification such as positive or negative, present or absent. The latter is called binary form (4, 6, 7).

DEFINITIONS

True positive (TP) Number of sick subjects correctly classified by the test, the positivity in disease.

False positive (FP) Number of subjects free of disease misclassified by the test, an error of commission.

True negative (TN) Number of subjects free of disease correctly classified by the test, the negativity in health.

False negative (FN) Number of sick subjects misclassified by the test, an error of omission.

Accuracy The degree of agreement between an observation and its true value determined by a superior method.

Precision The extent to which a series of observations agrees with one another.

Sensitivity Percent positivity in disease, the frequency of true positives, the true positive ratio expressed as a percentage.

$$\text{Sensitivity} = \frac{\text{true positives}}{\text{all sick patients}} \times 100$$

$$\text{Sensitivity} = \frac{\text{TP}}{\text{TP} + \text{FN}} \times 100$$

Specificity Percent negativity in health, the frequency of true negatives, the true negative ratio expressed as a percentage.

$$\text{Specificity} = \frac{\text{true negatives}}{\text{all subjects free of disease}} \times 100$$

$$\text{Specificity} = \frac{\text{TN}}{\text{TN} + \text{FP}} \times 100$$

False positive ratio The proportion of positive tests in all patients without disease.

$$\text{FP ratio} = \frac{\text{FP}}{\text{FP} + \text{TN}}$$

False negative ratio The proportion of negative results in all patients with disease.

$$\text{FN ratio} = \frac{\text{FN}}{\text{FN} + \text{TP}}$$

Predictive value of a positive result Percentage of positive results that are true positives, the probability of disease.

$$\text{Predictive value } (+) = \frac{\text{TP}}{\text{TP} + \text{FP}} \times 100$$

Predictive value of a negative result Percentage of nagative results that are true negatives, the probability of no disease.

$$\text{Predictive value } (-) = \frac{\text{TN}}{\text{FN} + \text{TN}} \times 100$$

Efficiency Percentage correctly classified by the test. Sometimes called the accuracy of the test, the ratio of correct outcomes to all outcomes expressed as a percentage.

$$\text{Efficiency} = \frac{\text{TP} + \text{TN}}{\text{TP} + \text{FP} + \text{FN} + \text{TN}} \times 100$$

Likelihood ratio The ratio of the true positive ratio to the false positive ratio.

$$\text{Likelihood} = \frac{\text{TP}}{\text{TP} + \text{FN}} \quad \frac{\text{FP} + \text{TN}}{\text{FP}}$$

Binary form results are neatly organized in a decision table which is a fourfold table of the results of two sets, each having a binary outcome:

Test result	Disease present	Disease absent
Positive	True positives	Error of commission
Negative	Error of omission	True negatives

or, using abbreviations:

Test result	Disease present	Disease absent	Totals
Positive	TP	FP	TP + FP
Negative	FN	TN	FN + TN
Totals	TP + FN	FP + TN	TP + FN + FP + TN

Since tests are either positive or negative, the TP ratio + FN ratio = 1.0

and the FP ratio + TN ratio = 1.0. The following example shows the use of decision tables. The results of radioisotope scans of the liver were studied (6), showing either disease or no disease on pathological examination. Of 344 tests TP = 231, FN = 27, FP = 32, and TN = 54. In the following decision table the ratios appear in brackets.

Liver Scans

Test	Disease	No disease	Totals
Positive	231 [0.9]	32 [0.37]	263
Negative	27 [0.1]	54 [0.63]	81
Totals	258	86	344

Sensitivity = 90%.
Specificity = 63%.
Predictive value of a positive result = 88%.
Predictive value of a negative result = 67%.
Efficiency = 83%.

Numerical Results

When numerical results are received from a test performed in a laboratory, the problem is to know what is considered normal for that test in the local population; an understanding of the derivation of the normal range is needed. A large group of observations is required to establish the normal range. Numerical results extend on a continuous range, part of which is considered normal because it includes the results from the majority of people. By convention the lowest 2.5% and the highest 2.5% of the numerical results is considered abnormal, the remaining 95% normal. The lowest and highest of these normal results define the normal range.

If the results follow the normal distribution, which is the familiar bell-shaped curve, the 95% range can be estimated in a more precise way by using the mean plus or minus two standard deviations (mean ±2d). In some experiments the definition of normalcy might be more restrictive, including less than 95%, or less restrictive, including more than 95% as the cutoff point for normals. For instance, if the mean ±1.6d is used, 90% is considered normal, whereas if the mean ±3.3d is used, 99.9% is considered normal (Figure 13).

Numerical results can be reduced to binary results by classifying them as normal or abnormal using the above concept of normalcy. Once the results are in binary form, a decision table can be made and specificity and sensitivity can be calculated. Depending upon the choice of the percentage of the results considered normal, the specificity and sensitivity change, since a different ratio of results is classified as true positive, true negative, false positive, and false negative. A series of normal ranges may be chosen and for each the specificity and sensitivity ratios calculated. These may be plotted as a graph

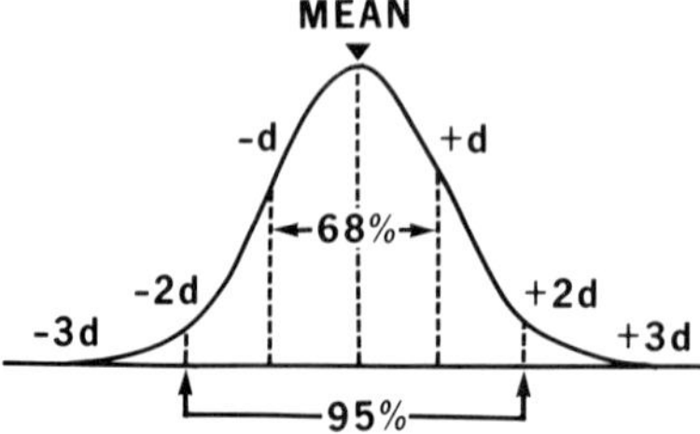

Figure 13 Frequency distribution curve. d is a standard deviation; +d and −d incorporate two standard deviations, or 68%; and +2d and −2d incorporate four standard deviations, or 95% of the total.

called the receiver-operating characteristic curve (Figure 14). From this curve one can choose a reasonable combination of low specificity and high sensitivity. The normal range that produces this combination is accepted as the cutoff point for normalcy. Having established the normal range, the numerical results are reduced to binary form, normal or abnormal.

Similarly one could construct a receiver-operating characteristic curve for the percentage of results considered abnormal for a particular test of a particular disease. From this receiver-operating characteristic curve one can establish the abnormal range for the test. Thus the test result may be diagnostic, showing health or disease, or nondiagnostic if the result falls outside both ranges.

An abnormal test result must be considered only with full knowledge of the normal range. Furthermore the relationship of the test result to the abnormal range for that test should be considered. Often, inexperienced physicians accept slightly elevated or slightly depressed results as significant,

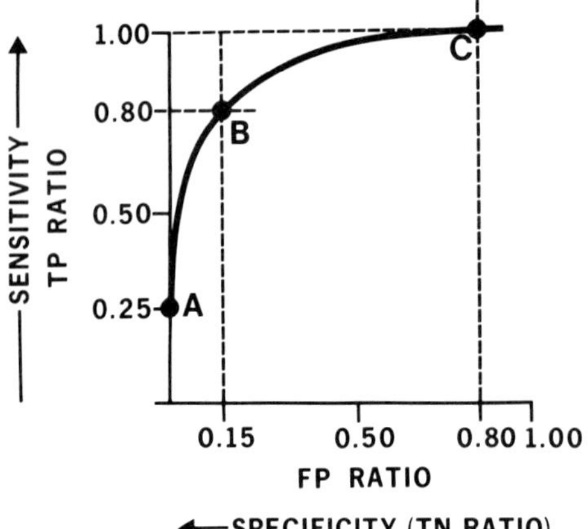

Figure 14 Hypothetical receiver-operating characteristic curve. At A the test has poor sensitivity (TP ratio = 0.25) but high specificity (TN ratio = 1.0 because FP ratio = 0). At C the test has high sensitivity (TP ratio = 1.0) but poor specificity (TN ratio = 0.2 because FP ratio = 0.8). The cutoff for a test might be point B because the sensitivity is good (TP ratio = 0.8) and the specificity also is good (TN ratio = 0.85 because the FP ratio = 0.15) (6, 7).

whereas they may be irrelevant. In every case the clinician should consider abnormal results only in relation to the patient's condition. When results are inappropriate, immediate evidence from clinical observation usually outweighs mediate evidence from laboratory tests.

If the conventional mean ±2d is taken as the normal range and each of a group of normal subjects has 10 multiphasic tests performed, half of these subjects would have one abnormal test result, a sobering thought.

REFERENCES

1. Asher R: Richard Asher Talking Sense. London: Pitman, 1972.
2. Botsford TW, Wilson RE: The Acute Abdomen, 2d ed. Philadelphia: Saunders, 1977.
3. Fisher MS: The analysis of survey abdominal radiographs in intestinal ileus. Weekly Radiology Science Update 1:5, 1976.
4. Galen RS, Gambino SR: Beyond Normality: The Predictive Value and Efficiency of Medical Diagnoses. New York: Wiley, 1975.
5. Gough MH, Gear MWL: The Plain X-Ray in the Diagnosis of the Acute Abdomen. Oxford: Blackwell, 1971.
6. McNeil BJ, Adelstein SJ: Determining the value of diagnostic and screening tests. J Nucl Med 17:439–448, 1976.
7. McNeil BJ, Keeler E, Adelstein SJ: Primer on certain elements of medical decision making. N Engl J Med 293:211–215, 1975.
8. Tyrer JH, Eadie MJ: The Astute Physician. Amsterdam: Elsevier, 1976.

Chapter 7

Pain from Various Organs

The quality of pain arising in the abdomen, pelvis, or chest may be so characteristic that the disturbance causing the pain can be immediately identified. Often however the type of pain, its distribution, and its other characteristics need to be known to reach a diagnosis. An understanding of the characteristics of pain that may be distinctive for organs or disease processes is necessary for proper evaluation of abdominal pain. Pain as it is usually encountered in both health and disease is described below for abdominal organs and for other organs that may bear consideration in differential diagnosis of abdominal pain. The latter include the pelvic urogenital organs, retroperitoneal urinary organs, aorta, the back, chest wall, lungs, and heart.

ESOPHAGUS

Distension of the esophagus by inflation of a swallowed balloon produces visceral pain. Pollard and Bloomfield (34) and Jones (17, 18) studied this pain in human volunteers and found that the pain was usually felt in the front, in the midline, at levels closely corresponding to the level of the balloon, but rarely in the back. Their volunteers found that the pain of distension was felt at all levels from the sternomanubrial joint to the xiphoid process. Sensory innervation of the esophagus is segmental so that the level of pain corresponds with the level of stimulation in most instances.

Many familiar stimuli cause pain in the esophagus. Everybody has felt the discomfort of swallowing fluids that are too hot or too cold and boluses of food that are too large. In addition to thermal and mechanical stimulation, electrical and chemical stimulation by cautery, acids, and other chemicals provokes pain. Radiological examination during stimulation shows contraction of the esophagus, often at the level of stimulation, and reverse peristalsis (17). Prompt disappearance of pain follows removal of the stimulus. Although pain is produced by muscle contraction, and antispasmodics provide some relief, visceral pain from the esophagus is frequently felt in the absence of evidence of smooth muscle contraction. Cold tends to stimulate smooth muscle contraction; moderate heat tends to relax smooth muscle.

Deep or somatic pain from the esophagus is difficult to differentiate from visceral pain by quality alone. However, somatic pain which may be caused by inflammation or infiltration may be felt in the back at the level of the lesion, whereas visceral pain is rarely referred to the back. When pain from the esophagus is severe, regional intercostal muscles contract because of stimulation through spinal reflex arcs. In turn the muscle spasm causes restriction of inspiration, which results in a sensation of tightness or constriction resembling the distress of angina pectoris or myocardial infarction. Spasmodic contraction of the inferior constrictor of the pharynx, particularly the cricopharyngeus muscle, is thought to be the anatomical basis for globus hystericus, the sensation of a ball in the throat.

The nerves of the esophagus are derived from the vagus or 10th cranial nerves and the upper six thoracic nerves (29, 43). Pain may be felt anteriorly in the midline from the suprasternal notch to the epigastrium. Proximal spread occurs readily if the pain is severe. Pain in the suprasternal notch may be caused by irritation of the esophagus at that level or at its lower end. Spread may occur to the inner side of the arms, the sides of the neck, the jaws, the ear, and the side of the face; all of these are in the distribution of afferents that run though the branches of the cervical sympathetic ganglia and the branches of the vagus nerves. However, in most instances the pain is a deep thoracic discomfort at the level of stimulation. The most common referral is from the lower end of the esophagus to the suprasternal region. Evidence that the vagus nerves carry some of the afferent fibers from the esophagus is the discovery that pain from the esophagus can persist after transection of the spinal cord at the fifth cervical level, after high spinal anesthesia, after resection of the splanchnic nerves, and after resection of the thoracic sympathetic ganglia (11, 18, 35, 36, 40). The types and distribution of pain from the esophagus are summarized as follows:

Sensory innervation: Cervical and thoracic splanchnic branches (T1-6) and vagus nerves (X), esophageal plexus

Visceral pain: Central chest, close to the level of irritation

Somatic pain: Central chest, close to the level of irritation

Referred pain: (*a*) Midline in the back close to the level of irritation, (*b*) lower end of the esophagus to the suprasternal notch

Heartburn

Heartburn or pyrosis is a burning sensation felt deep to the lower sternum. By far the most common stimulus is regurgitated acid gastric contents. Acid gastric juice containing bile is a stronger stimulus than acid without bile. Duodenal juice containing bile and pancreatic secretion is mildly alkaline and may cause heartburn after operations on the stomach or in achlorhydric patients. The intensity of heartburn is always greater in the presence of esophagitis, but esophagitis is not necessary for heartburn. Heartburn is similar to the pain of peptic ulcer disease and is a superficial type of pain. It is midline, poorly localized, and often associated with increased tension in the muscles of the esophageal wall.

The lowermost circular muscle fibers of the esophagus comprise the lower esophageal sphincter. This sphincter is one of the important mechanisms preventing reflux from the stomach, the other being the intra-abdominal position of the lower esophagus, which is subject to positive intra-abdominal pressure. Sliding hiatus hernia is often associated with heartburn, but heartburn can occur with a lax lower esophageal sphincter and no hiatus hernia. Similarly a patient having a sliding hiatus hernia may have an effective lower esophageal sphincter and no heartburn in spite of the fact that the lower esophagus lies in the thorax. Heartburn is worse with obesity, tight clothing such as corsets and belts, lying flat, bending forward, and stooping. Alcohol aggravates heartburn by increasing gastric acidity and decreasing the tone of the lower esophageal sphincter. Excessive air swallowing, large meals, and physical straining promote reflux. Dysphagia associated with heartburn may be caused by spasm or stricture in the lower esophagus.

Antacids in liquid form provide relief from heartburn within a few seconds of swallowing; the tablet form is less effective. In addition to coating the lower esophagus antacids reduce the acidity of gastric juice, thereby providing more lasting relief. Antispasmodics may provide some relief from heartburn but are more likely to aggravate it by allowing more gastric regurgitation.

Diffuse Esophageal Spasm

Diffuse esophageal spasm is a motility disorder of the esophagus characterized by intermittent dysphagia and pain. Esophagograms show hyperactive tertiary spasmodic contractions and absence of normal peristalsis in the lower half of the esophagus. Cold liquids, reflux of gastric juice, and stress precipitate and aggravate this condition. Steady, severe lower thoracic and upper abdominal visceral pain suggests either diffuse esophageal spasm, myocardial ischemia, or biliary colic. When severe, there is painful contraction of intercostal muscles, a feeling of suffocation, and proximal spread of pain to the neck, arms, and face.

Spontaneous Rupture

If a patient vomits forcefully after a large meal, especially after drinking alcohol in excess, and develops severe thoracic pain and shock, spontaneous rupture of the esophagus is suspected. Examination may reveal a left hydropneumothorax. This condition is rare, serious, and requires emergency surgical care.

Esophageal Stricture

Obstruction of the esophagus may be associated with pain on swallowing. Steady pain may occur from the inflammation of a penetrating peptic ulcer of the esophagus or infiltration of an esophageal malignant tumor to nearby nerves, blood vessels, or bone. Steady, unrelenting deep chest pain and back pain with dysphagia suggest infiltrating carcinoma of the esophagus.

STOMACH

Rapid distension of the stomach produces visceral pain as everyone who has gulped foods or fluids in large quantity knows. Much of the information concerning the sensibility of the stomach has resulted from observations on human subjects having large gastrocutaneous fistulas. In 1825 William Beaumont observed the gastric functions of his patient Alexis St. Martin (1). In 1942 Wolf and Wolff reported many observations on their patient Tom (46). Wolf and Wolff (45) have shown that pain of considerable intensity is produced by mechanical or chemical stimulation of the stomach when it is inflamed, congested, or edematous. Pinching normal gastric mucosa caused no pain. Normal hydrochloric acid, one-tenth normal sodium hydroxide, 50–95% alcohol, or 1/30 suspension of mustard did not cause pain in healthy mucosa. When the stomach was inflamed, these stimuli evoked intense pain.

The stomach becomes sensitive as it becomes congested. Stress is known to cause hyperemia of the gastric mucosa. Clearly there is a psychosomatic mechanism for pain from the stomach. In a physiological sense the sensitivity of congestion seems to resemble primary cutaneous hyperalgesia and perhaps hyperalgesia secondary to inflammation (36).

Visceral pain is the main type of pain from the stomach. When inflammations and infiltrations extend beyond the gastric serosa to parietal peritoneum, somatic pain is felt. Referred pain and pain from regional muscle contraction rarely accompany visceral pain from the stomach. Extension of inflammation from the stomach or infiltration of a neoplasm outside the stomach causes somatic pain, peritoneal irritation, and muscle guarding.

The greater part of sensory innervation reaches the stomach by way of the fifth to ninth thoracic spinal nerves through the greater splanchnic nerves, thoracic splanchnic branches, and the celiac ganglia. Most authors believe that the vagus nerves also carry pain fibers to the stomach. Vagal stimulation during operations under local anesthesia causes visceral pain in the midepigastrium. Visceral pain from the abdomen can be felt by quadriplegics who are known to have complete transection of the cervical spinal cord (6, 10, 14, 16). Duodenal ulcer pain relief after truncal vagotomy cannot be taken as evidence for this belief because this pain is also eliminated by parietal cell or proximal gastric vagotomy; the vagotomy must be assumed to eliminate the cause for the pain rather than to interrupt pain pathways.

Pain from the stomach is distributed as shown below:

Sensory innervation: Greater splanchnic nerves (T5–T9) and vagus nerves (X), celiac plexus
Visceral pain: Midepigastrium
Somatic pain: Midepigastrium, left upper quadrant
Referred pain: Rare

Peptic Ulcer

Peptic ulcer pain can arise from ulceration of the duodenum, stomach, lower esophagus, or jejunum adjacent to a gastrojejunostomy. Many clinical and experimental observations show that acidity is the immediate precipitating factor. Acid in the ulcer causes pain, and neutralizing or removing the acid from the vicinity relieves the pain of uncomplicated peptic ulcer. Local smooth muscle contraction precipitated by acid is another factor because intravenous antispasmodics can provide relief. Hyperperistalsis in the absence of acid does not evoke pain but acid without hyperperistalsis or sustained smooth muscle contraction does.

Duodenal Ulcer

The typical pain of duodenal ulcer disease, the only superficial type of pain arising from the small bowel, is described as a burning or gnawing discomfort typical of a continuous superficial pain. There is no clear explanation for this type of pain, but perhaps frequency and familiarity cause facilitation; or smooth muscle contraction, local congestion, and inflammation increase the sensitivity; or inflammation reaching the serosa causes superficial pain felt as part of parietal pain.

The most characteristic feature of duodenal ulcer pain is its daily rhythm corresponding to the concentration of acid in the ulcer. Pain is rarely felt on first awakening in the morning but appears about $1\frac{1}{2}$ hours after each meal and often immediately before the noon meal, the evening meal, or bedtime. Night pain may awaken the duodenal ulcer patient between midnight and four o'clock in the morning. The distress of uncomplicated duodenal ulcer disease is relieved within 5 to 15 minutes by the ingestion of milk, foods, or antacids. Vomiting brings about early relief. Any patient having epigastric discomfort with this rhythm must be suspected of having peptic ulcer disease. In fact, pain with this characteristic rhythm dictates the management of these patients in spite of nondiagnostic X-rays or endoscopic examination. Exacerbation of the pain in the spring and autumn is the rule and remains unexplained. Ulcer management must include measures that give relief and avoid those that precipitate or increase this pain. A change in attitude and behavior and the avoidance of tobacco, alcohol, and irritating foods and fluids form the essence of an ulcer regimen. A reduced pace of work and more diversion from the stresses of life are more important than dietary changes. Regular meals may be more important than the type of food. The importance of acidity cannot be denied: duodenal ulcer disease does not occur in those who are achlorhydric, and ulcers heal faster when gastric acidity is greatly reduced.

Penetrating Duodenal Ulcer Penetration of a posterior wall duodenal ulcer is suspected when back pain is felt in addition to the typical epigastric distress. As a rule pain felt in the epigastrium becomes more severe, more constant, and less easily relieved by food and antacid as penetration occurs. The back pain is dull, deep, and constant. It is a referred pain which, as a rule, is not associated with muscle contraction or tenderness in the back. Penetration of a duodenal ulcer may be associated with a slight increase in concentration of pancreatic amylase in the serum.

Perforation Perforation of a duodenal ulcer usually begins suddenly and dramatically. There may or may not be preceding duodenal ulcer pain. Back pain preceding perforation is very rare since only anterior ulcers perforate; posterior duodenal ulcers penetrate and cause bleeding. Duodenal ulcer pain may increase in frequency and severity preceding perforation. A rapid onset of very severe, steady abdominal pain accompanied by severe involuntary reflex abdominal wall muscle guarding means an intraperitoneal perforation. Duodenal contents are very irritating, and the rigidity of abdominal wall muscles is complete or boardlike. Any movement increases pain—the patient lies immobile and frightened, breathing shallowly with the upper thorax rather than the lower thorax and diaphragm. The peritonitis is severe, and referred pain is often felt on the tops of the shoulders from irritation of the central diaphragm.

Occasionally free spillage of duodenal contents is less rapid and more localized causing a less severe degree of peritonitis. Duodenal juice may run down the right side of the peritoneal cavity causing right flank and right lower quadrant peritonitis that suggests appendicitis. Free air in the peritoneal cavity confirms the diagnosis of a perforation, although X-rays are not necessary when the clinical picture is typical.

Other Complications Pain is relieved when hemorrhage from a duodenal ulcer occurs since blood is a buffer of acid. Similarly pain is not a problem with pyloric obstruction because scarring occludes the pylorus and acid gastric juice can no longer reach the ulcer region.

Benign Gastric Ulcer

Gastric ulcer is difficult to distinguish from duodenal ulcer by history alone. There is a tendency for the pain of gastric ulcer to appear earlier after eating, often within the first hour. Patients believe that eating causes pain; so they become afraid of eating and lose their appetites. Gastritis in the presence of gastric ulcer increases anorexia. Some patients find that vomiting relieves the pain promptly and some induce vomiting. Nocturnal hypersecretion and pain rarely occur in the absence of pyloric stenosis. The pain of gastric ulcer tends to be relieved earlier but for a shorter period of time by antacid, milk, and most foods. However these differences are unreliable for differentiating duodenal from gastric ulcer. Prepyloric gastric ulcer and pyloric channel ulcer have the characteristics and behavior of duodenal ulcers except that ulcers in these regions may be malignant.

Gastritis

Although the pain of gastritis resembles the pain of duodenal or gastric ulcer, it is more persistent and less readily relieved by antacids, food, or fluids. It is frequently accompanied by nausea and vomiting, but vomiting does not afford much relief. Because alcohol is the common cause of gastritis, it is often accompanied by pancreatitis.

Postgastrectomy Pain Syndromes

There are five pain syndromes that may follow operations on the stomach or duodenum: (*a*) Steady midepigastric pain appearing soon after the beginning of a meal and subsiding shortly afterwards may be caused by too small a gastric pouch following gastrectomy. (*b*) Right upper abdominal steady severe pain following a meal relieved by vomiting of bile is characteristic of the postgastrectomy afferent loop syndrome. This syndrome may follow a gastrojejunostomy when the pylorus is divided or stenosed. (*c*) Crampy periumbilical pain occurring 10–20 minutes after eating may follow any operation that changes or eliminates the pyloric sphincter. It is caused by rapid passage of gastric contents into the small bowel, the dumping syndrome. (*d*) One of the most common postgastrectomy complaints is pain accompanied by nothing more than distal gastritis, currently called reflux alkaline or bile gastritis. Medical therapy is difficult and disappointing. Surgical diversion of bile away from the stomach is safe only when the vagotomy is complete or a high gastrectomy has been performed. (*e*) Volvulus, intussusception, or internal hernia are rare complications that cause pain by small bowel obstruction following operations on the stomach.

Gastric Neoplasm

When tumors are confined to the stomach wall there may be no symptoms other than anorexia. Some patients have ulcer-type distress before eating, whereas others have steady discomfort for a short period after eating. When the tumor infiltrates or causes pressure outside the stomach wall, the pain becomes relentlessly steady in the epigastrium and in the back.

Other Gastric Diseases

Volvulus of the stomach produces severe upper abdominal steady pain, vomiting, and shock. Strangulated paraesophageal hiatus hernia produces severe left chest pain, vomiting, and shock. In fact these conditions may occur together since the stomach undergoes rotation while rolling into the chest through a large paraesophageal opening in the diaphragm.

The diagnosis of peptic ulcer, gastritis, or gastric neoplasm is established by inspection and biopsy if the lesion can be seen through a gastroscope. X-ray appearances may be diagnostic or highly suggestive. A typical peptic ulcer history alone is sufficient for a provisional diagnosis and an ulcer regimen.

LIVER

The parenchyma of the liver is insensitive; however, the capsule of the liver is sensitive, and rapid enlargement of the liver causes steady right upper abdominal pain. Inflammation and infiltration in the liver produce right upper quadrant pain that may be aggravated by breathing. The liver is supplied by the 5th to 9th thoracic nerves by way of the greater splanchnic nerves and celiac ganglia. The liver is in contact with parietal peritoneum supplied by the right 6th to 12th thoracic nerves, the left 6th and 7th thoracic nerves, and both phrenic nerves. Gradual enlargement of the liver occurs without pain. Occasionally inflammation reaching the capsule of the liver produces irritation of parietal peritoneum and pain on breathing associated with an audible friction rub. This pain must be differentiated from the pain of right-sided pleurisy. Hepatitis and congestive hepatomegaly cause steady, dull right upper quadrant abdominal pain, and the liver is tender. Fatty infiltration, neoplasms, and cirrhosis seldom cause pain and tenderness.

GALLBLADDER AND BILE DUCTS

Balloon distension of the gallbladder through a cholecystostomy wound produces midline, steady epigastric pain. In spite of its name biliary colic is steady. Rapid distension of the bile ducts by T-tube injection or by endoscopic retrograde cannulation produces biliary colic indistinguishable from the biliary colic arising from the gallbladder. Rapid distension of the gallbladder or bile ducts is the stimulus for biliary colic; slow distension is pain free. When a gallstone becomes impacted in the cystic duct, rapid distension occurs because of secretion by the gallbladder mucosa. When a gallstone suddenly blocks the lower common bile duct, secretion of bile and possibly pancreatic juice rapidly distends the ducts and causes biliary colic. Smooth muscle is sparse in the walls of the ducts, and its contraction probably plays a very minor role; antispasmodics afford little relief.

As with other viscera arising from the foregut, the biliary system receives visceral innervation through both greater splanchnic nerves. Because of bilateral innervation, the brain interprets biliary colic as arising in the midline. Biliary colic is a steady pain and generally lasts from 20 minutes to several hours. As a rule biliary colic occurs usually only once in 24 hours. Rarely two short attacks may occur in one day, but not three. When biliary colic is severe the pain may radiate to the back, usually in the midline in the interscapular region. It may also be associated with severe contraction of the lower intercostal muscles, which in turn causes pain around the lower chest. Inspiration is restricted and the patient describes a smothering tightness, a feeling of a weight on the chest, or the feeling of a tight band around the lower ribs. Severe biliary colic is similar to the distress of myocardial ischemia or diffuse esophageal spasm. There is no shoulder-top pain in uncomplicated biliary colic; so it is doubtful that phrenic nerve fibers reach the gallbladder or bile ducts.

Following are the types and distribution of pain from the gallbladder and bile ducts:

Sensory innervation: Greater splanchnic nerves (T5-9) and vagus nerves (X), celiac plexus

Visceral pain: Midepigastrium

Somatic pain: Right upper quadrant over the fundus of the gallbladder

Referred pain: Interscapular region (associated with biliary colic), inferior angle of the right scapula, right shoulder top from irritation of the central part of the right diaphragm

Acute cholecystitis may be preceded by biliary colic. When biliary colic associated with cystic duct obstruction lasts four hours or longer, inflammation and infection have developed in the gallbladder and the diagnosis of biliary colic should be changed to acute cholecystitis. As this happens the right upper quadrant somatic pain of acute cholecystitis begins and becomes more severe than the disappearing midline visceral pain of biliary colic. The timing of these changes can vary with the severity of the infection in the gallbladder. The inflammation in the wall of the gallbladder spreads rapidly to the serosa and stimulates the parietal peritoneum. Parietal peritoneal irritation often produces a referred pain at the inferior angle of the right scapula. Irritation of the inferior surface of the right diaphragm causes right shoulder-top pain. For unknown reasons approximately 1 patient in 10 complains also of left upper quadrant pain, and 1 in 25 having acute cholecystitis and normal serum amylase complains initially of left upper quadrant pain alone. As generally happens once the right upper quadrant tenderness develops, these patients complain of pain at the site of the tenderness; few mention left-sided abdominal pain thereafter. Occasionally hyperesthesia and hyperalgesia can be demonstrated in the right sixth to ninth thoracic dermatomes.

Guarding of abdominal wall muscles is expected with acute cholecystitis: in mild cases it is confined to the right upper quadrant; in severe cases it is severe in the upper quadrants, moderate in the lower quadrants, and severe in the lower intercostal muscles on both sides. Movement produces pain so that breathing is confined to the upper chest, and the lower chest and diaphragm are kept as still as possible. The tensely contracted abdominal wall and lower thoracic intercostal muscles soon become painful and tender.

A stone may suddenly become impacted in the lower common bile duct and cause biliary colic. If this pain lasts several hours there is increasing risk of infection. Acute cholangitis is recognized by right upper quadrant abdominal pain, often radiating to the back; chills; fever, which is often high and intermittent; and obstructive jaundice.

In summary, gallstone disease can produce all types of pain and all of the physiological phenomena associated with pain. Biliary colic is a visceral pain that, when severe, is associated with reflex muscle contraction and radiation of the pain to the back, to the interscapular region or occasionally to the inferior angle of the right scapula. The pain of acute cholecystitis is parietal pain over the gallbladder associated with local peritoneal irritation, and referred pain to the inferior angle of the right scapula and to the top of the right shoulder. Intercostal muscle contraction and abdominal wall guarding are expected, and soon these muscles become painful and tender. Tightness of these muscles produces a sensation of suffocation or tightness in the chest. As with appendicitis, if the pain of acute cholecystitis seems to improve unexpectedly, beware. The gallbladder wall may undergo gangrene, and perforation may be imminent. Paracholecystic abscess or diffuse peritonitis is the consequence of gangrene of the gallbladder. Acute cholangitis is characterized by right upper quadrant pain, chills, fever, and jaundice; it is not complicated by perforation but by septic shock and death.

Certain radiological investigations of the biliary system are sensitive and often diagnostic. These include oral cholecystography and percutaneous transhepatic, operative, and endoscopic retrograde cholangiography. When intravenous cholangiography is performed for at least two hours and tomograms are taken and studied with care, strong and usually diagnostic evidence can be obtained.

PANCREAS

Visceral pain from the pancreas may be produced by rapid injection of fluid into the pancreatic duct through a catheter left in place after operation or inserted by endoscopic retrograde cannulation of the pancreatic duct. Visceral pain from the pancreas is steady, midline, and midepigastric. Because the pancreas is a foregut structure, there is steady visceral pain similar to biliary colic. It is believed that visceral pain from the pancreas is carried by both greater splanchnic nerves. However, somatic pain is more important in pancreatic disease, and the somatic nerve supply is the first lumbar nerve. The first lumbar nerve has little representation in the anterior abdominal wall muscles, another reason for the late onset of the signs of peritoneal irritation in pancreatitis. Eventually intraperitoneal exudate and blood stimulate lower thoracic nerves and cause peritoneal irritation and signs of peritonitis. Pain from the pancreas is distributed as follows:

Sensory innervation: Greater splanchnic nerves (T5–9) and vagus nerves (X), celiac plexus

Visceral pain: Midepigastrium

Somatic pain: Midepigastrium or on the right or left over the pancreas

Referred pain: Midline of the back at the level of the first lumbar vertebra

In acute pancreatitis surrounding structures are irritated early so that somatic pain occurs early. The pancreas is a retroperitoneal organ; so parietal nerve stimulation is expected, and pain is referred to the back in the region of the spine of the first lumbar vertebra. Signs of peritoneal irritation do not appear early. One of the characteristics of acute pancreatitis is that the severity of the pain seems out of proportion to the physical signs. Often patients are suspected of being malingerers or narcotic addicts. It is likely that these characteristics are caused by the retroperitoneal position of the pancreas.

Much of the pain and vascular collapse in acute pancreatitis is caused by stimulation and absorption by the peritoneum of the intraperitoneal fluid containing vasoactive polypeptides. Evidence for this is the fact that removal of this fluid by peritoneal lavage provides remarkable relief from pain and reversal of circulatory collapse. The extent of the pathological changes in the pancreas is not influenced by peritoneal lavage. Whenever the symptoms and signs of acute pancreatitis persist beyond a week, be aware of a possible pseudocyst or pancreatic abscess.

Tragically pain is not felt early in the development of carcinoma of the pancreas. Later in the disease steady pain appears and is characteristically unrelenting and deep in the midline of the epigastrium. The pain is later felt in the back at the spine of the first lumbar vertebra. Paroxysmal pain is unusual. Some patients gain a little relief by sitting, leaning forward, and supporting the upper abdomen with their folded forearms. Obstructive jaundice caused by carcinoma of the pancreas is more often painful than not. The early pain in pancreatic carcinoma is a visceral pain, and the likely cause is pancreatic duct obstruction. Later pain is caused by infiltration of perineural tissues. Finally invasion of tumor to structures outside the pancreas and pressure from metastasis are responsible for pain.

Because the pain of pancreatic cancer may be mild yet constant without any diagnostic signs or tests, some patients are poorly handled by their physicians. The constancy of the pain makes them chronic complainers. Failure of these patients to respond to tranquilizers, group therapy, or physiotherapy should lead one to review the diagnosis and consider the possibility of a deep malignancy such as carcinoma of the pancreas. Recent onset of diabetes mellitus with epigastric pain should prompt intensive investigations for carcinoma of the pancreas.

Radiological investigations of the pancreas remain imprecise with a number of false negatives and false positives. Endoscopic retrograde pancreatography and arteriography are diagnostic occasionally. Computerized axial tomography demonstrates the pancreas and shows an increase in size. Isotope scans have been of limited value in the diagnosis of pancreatic neoplasm. Ultrasonography has proven useful in identifying pancreatic cysts, pseudocysts, and masses.

Elevation of serum amylase concentration more than five times the upper limit of normal is considered diagnostic of acute pancreatitis, but the level does not indicate the severity of the attack. A decreased concentration of serum calcium indicates severe acute pancreatitis. The concentration of amylase in the urine or pleural or peritoneal fluid can be highly suggestive if not diagnostic of pancreatitis.

SPLEEN

The parenchyma of the spleen is insensitive; the capsule is sensitive to rapid stretching and inflammation; and the adjacent parietal peritoneum is sensitive to the irritation of blood or inflammation of the splenic capsule. Visceral pain from the spleen may be felt during splenoportography when percutaneous splenic puncture is done under local anesthesia. Rapid injection of contrast solution may cause vague epigastric pain.

Abdominal injury complicated by rupture of the spleen causes pain resulting from the irritating effects of blood in the peritoneal cavity. Subcapsular hematoma of the spleen does not cause discomfort sufficiently typical to permit diagnosis. Delayed rupture of a subcapsular hematoma may occur hours to months after trauma and is characterized by unexpected onset of pain caused by intraperitoneal hemorrhage. Irritation of parietal nerves in the region of the spleen commonly produces pain on the top of the left shoulder. The diseased spleen is more prone to rupture, especially the large spleen of malaria or the soft spleen of infectious mononucleosis, and in the latter case spontaneous rupture may occur.

Sudden, sharp somatic left upper quadrant pain may be caused by splenic infarcts. Splenic infarcts may be caused by arterial emboli from bacterial endocarditis, myocardial infarction, atrial fibrillation, or an aneurysm. Infarcts may be caused by splenic arterial thrombosis secondary to leukemia, sickle-cell disease, and polycythemia vera. Focal infarcts occur in acute septicemia.

Dull, aching left-sided abdominal pain may be caused by massive splenomegaly. Traction on the peritoneal attachments of the large spleen is believed to be the mechanism.

SMALL INTESTINE

Before long, everyone becomes well acquainted with crampy abdominal pain. Cramps or colic are recognized as the response of the intestine to infection, spoiled foods, and laxatives. Excessive motor activity of the midgut, that is, the duodenum beyond the duodenal papilla, the jejunum, the ileum, the cecum, and the ascending and transverse sections of the large intestine, causes periumbilical crampy pain. Distension of the small bowel by balloon tubes inserted through the mouth or nose or through enterostomy stomata demonstrates that distension is the stimulus for contraction of the wall of the bowel (17). Rapid distension of these balloons produces immediate pain. Slow distension of the intestine neither causes pain nor stimulates muscle contraction.

Although crampy abdominal pain is the most frequent pain from the small intestine, the small bowel can give rise to steady visceral pain, which is thought to be caused by hypoxia from an impaired mesenteric circulation. Steady pain may also arise from a distended segment that is unable to empty, such as an obstructed closed loop of bowel.

Visceral pain from the midgut is carried by visceral afferent fibers that arise from the 10th thoracic to the 1st lumbar spinal nerves and run through the superior mesenteric ganglion. Some visceral afferent fibers from the midgut are carried in the vagus nerves, evidenced by the ability to feel visceral pain from the midgut after bilateral splanchnic nerve resection (3), and by quadriplegics who have proven complete cord transection above the level of the first thoracic nerve (6, 10, 14, 16). Resection of the celiac and superior mesenteric ganglia and their branches interrupts these visceral pain pathways (39, 42, 44).

Somatic pain from the midgut can be caused by irritation of the root of the mesentery. When traction, inflammation, infiltration, or other irritation reaches the parietal peritoneum, somatic pain is felt and local tenderness and muscle guarding occur. Occasionally hyperalgesia and hyperesthesia can be demonstrated in the stimulated dermatomes.

Types and distribution of pain from the small intestine are presented below:

Sensory innervation: Thoracic and lumbar splanchnic nerves (T10–L1) and vagus nerves (X), superior mesenteric plexus
Visceral pain: Umbilical
Somatic pain: Over the site of the irritation
Referred pain: Very rare

Mechanical Small Bowel Obstruction

Crampy periumbilical abdominal pain, distension of the abdomen, obstipation, and nausea and vomiting are characteristic of obstruction of the small bowel distal to the duodenal papilla or the large bowel proximal to the splenic flexure. The higher the level of the obstruction, the earlier the onset of vomiting. As a rule the shorter the free interval between cramps the higher the obstruction. One or two bowel movements may occur after the onset of obstruction, but once the bowel beyond the obstruction has emptied there is no further passage of feces or gas by rectum. Periumbilical cramps, abdominal distension, and diarrhea suggest incomplete obstruction of the midgut. The lower the level of intestinal obstruction, the earlier and the greater will be the distension. (See also Chapter 8.)

In typical small bowel obstruction each wave of pain is brief, usually lasting less than a minute and recurring every two to four minutes. There is little or no pain between the cramps. During the cramps the patient doubles up, often drawing the thighs up to the abdominal wall since supporting the abdomen seems to give some relief. Exaggerated peristaltic contractions produce loud intestinal sounds. Shortly accumulation of gas and fluid in the bowel proximal to the obstruction causes distension of the abdomen. With the patient lying supine the accumulated gas lies beneath the anterior abdominal wall and gives rise to tympanitic resonance on percussion. If the abdominal wall is thin and relaxed, peristaltic movements may be seen.

Acute Enteritis

Crampy abdominal pain preceded by nausea and vomiting, and followed by diarrhea is characteristic of acute enteritis. Abdominal distension is not a feature of acute enteritis, and incomplete bowel obstruction should be suspected when distension is found. In acute enteritis hyperactive peristaltic noises coinciding with the cramps are heard. Bowel sounds depend upon the presence of gas in the intestine. If there is no gas in the intestine, exaggerated bowel sounds are not heard despite the cramps (21). As a rule abdominal cramps are briefly relieved after passage of stool.

In malabsorption syndrome crampy abdominal pain may occur as well as distension, discomfort, and flatulence. Bowel movements are pale, frequent, loose, bulky, and offensive. The feces may float and stick to the inside of the toilet bowl requiring several flushings to wash them away. Abdominal cramps, bloating, and explosive diarrhea occur with lactose intolerance resulting from lactase deficiency. Volvulus may develop in the overfilled colon.

Other Causes

Poisoning from heavy metals such as lead, arsenic, or mercury causes abdominal cramps. Acute intermittent porphyria is associated with colic. Various laxatives, drugs, and hormones can induce intestinal cramps.

Intestinal Ischemia

Sudden onset of strangulation of the bowel may be caused by vascular occlusion by embolus or thrombosis or even low blood flow without thrombosis. Sudden or rapid onset of impairment of the circulation of the intestine causes rapid onset of steady visceral pain. The pain may be caused by ischemic anoxia or the accumulation of acid metabolites. The severity of the pain varies with the rapidity and degree of circulatory impairment. As a rule hemorrhage and edema occur in the bowel wall, initially in submucosa and later may extend through all layers. Fluid and often blood are lost into the lumen, and a watery or bloody diarrhea occurs. The syndrome of sudden or rapid onset of abdominal pain, soon followed by watery or bloody diarrhea, and vascular collapse characterizes mesenteric vascular occlusion. Early recognition of this syndrome is most important so that embolectomy or thrombectomy can be performed before gangrene supervenes. Bowel resection should be performed before perforation of gangrenous bowel occurs. (See also Chapter 8.)

Acute occlusion of the celiac artery is practically unknown. Chronic occlusion is an unlikely syndrome (28). Superior mesenteric artery occlusion may occur acutely with severe midgut steady pain, shock, and bloody diarrhea. The shock and pain are out of proportion to the degree of peritonitis so that pancreatitis is suspected. Slow occlusion may be pain free. Chronic impairment of circulation to the gut may cause malabsorption, weight loss, and postcibal pain, which has been called intestinal angina; it is a rare syndrome (38).

Acute occlusion of the inferior mesenteric artery may cause sudden hypogastric pain, shock, and bloody or watery diarrhea if the collateral circulatory link is impaired through marginal mesenteric vessels at the splenic flexure with branches of the superior mesenteric artery and at the recto-sigmoid with branches of the internal iliac arteries. Edema, congestion, and friability are recognized in the sigmoid colon by endoscopy and plain supine X-ray of the abdomen where gas in the sigmoid colon is outlined by the swollen mucosa.

Aortoiliac operations for aortic disease usually include division of the inferior mesenteric artery, which is usually well tolerated because of the progressive slow occlusion of the artery before the operation (8).

Early in arterial mesenteric occlusion, arteriography may be successful in demonstrating a block, and an emergency operation to open or bypass the artery may save the bowel. Otherwise resuscitation and other supportive measures are used to prepare the patient for resection of the gangrenous bowel.

Ischemia of the intestine may not be primary but secondary to mechanical intestinal obstruction, and then it is called intestinal strangulation. In this case there are symptoms and signs of mechanical obstruction complicated by severe, steady pain, vascular collapse, and tenderness over the strangulated intestine. Soon there is peritoneal irritation from blood in the peritoneal cavity. Sudden relief of the pain of strangulation may be appreciated by the patient but dreaded by the surgeon because this may bode perforation of gangrenous bowel and diffuse peritonitis. (See also Chapter 8.)

ACUTE PERITONITIS

Acute inflammation of the peritoneum causes severe, steady parietal abdominal pain. Intense stimulation of the peritoneum is caused by pus, gastric juice, intestinal contents, bile, blood, or other irritants in the peritoneal cavity. The intensity of the pain varies with the strength of the irritant and the extent of the peritoneal soiling. Pain is present in all parts of the abdomen as the irritant spreads diffusely throughout the peritoneal cavity. If the irritant is confined the pain is localized to the involved area. Fluid passes into the peritoneal cavity and the irritant becomes less concentrated. The displacement of fluid into the peritoneum, the severity of the pain, and the absorption of toxic products leads to hypovolemic shock. (See also Chapter 8.)

Acute peritonitis causes severe, steady abdominal pain that is associated with reflex contraction of the abdominal wall muscles. Diffuse peritonitis is associated with muscle guarding in all quadrants of the abdomen. Peritonitis confined to part of the abdomen may be associated with muscle guarding in that area and less severe or no guarding in other areas. The intensity of the peritoneal irritation determines the completeness of abdominal muscle contraction. In mild cases of peritonitis there may be little more than slight increase in the tone of abdominal wall muscles. In many cases of peritonitis the muscle contraction is obvious and sustained, but the abdominal wall can be indented by pressure. In most severe cases of acute peritonitis, the muscles remain in total contraction; they are rigid and indentation is impossible. Spread of this reflex muscle contraction may occur proximally to the lower intercostal muscles. Movement causes pain and muscle guarding prevents movement. The lower thoracic cage is held rigid by tense muscles and is not used for breathing. Similarly movement of the diaphragm is restricted. The patient lies still and uses only the upper thoracic muscles for breathing. As the trunk muscles remain in sustained contraction they become painful and tender, adding to the distress. Involuntary muscle guarding is the prime sign of peritoneal irritation.

Parietal peritoneal irritation of the posterior wall of the abdomen stimulates afferents in lumbar spinal nerves. Back pain, muscle contraction, and muscle tenderness may be found in the lumbar and lower thoracic regions in the back. Irritation of the anterior and lateral parietal peritoneal walls stimulates afferents in the lower seven thoracic spinal nerves. Pain and intercostal muscle guarding in these segments are common. Irritation of the central portion of the diaphragm causes shoulder-top pain through the phrenic nerve.

In regions of acute peritonitis, there is direct tenderness, tenderness to percussion, and local rebound tenderness. In other areas of the abdomen there is remote or referred tenderness and remote rebound tenderness. These signs help to determine the site of the most intense peritonitis and may suggest the cause. Hyperalgesia and hyperesthesia may be demonstrable within the stimulated dermatomes.

ACUTE APPENDICITIS

Acute appendicitis is the most common cause of acute peritonitis and is the most common urgent surgical condition of the abdomen. Any patient with diffuse abdominal pain followed by right lower quadrant pain and tenderness must be suspected of having acute appendicitis. Early diagnosis and treatment are essential to avoid mortality and morbidity.

The sequence of events in acute appendicitis is important. At the onset there is periumbilical midgut visceral pain, usually crampy but occasionally steady. Symptoms of gastrointestinal upset soon appear. There is anorexia, often nausea, and occasionally vomiting. Constipation is expected; diarrhea is unusual. Periumbilical visceral pain disappears as right lower quadrant somatic pain and tenderness appear. Signs of local or diffuse peritonitis make the diagnosis reasonably certain. Systemic signs such as fever, tachycardia, perspiration, and leukocytosis indicate the presence of infection.

Unfortunately variations in this typical sequence are common. Occasionally the early visceral pain is absent. If the periumbilical pain is severe and steady, the surgeon should suspect that the appendix is obstructed, undergoing distension, in which case there is a greater possibility of early gangrene and perforation. The patient may not have noticed or may deny anorexia or nausea. The site of the right lower quadrant somatic pain varies with the position of the appendix. Once tenderness develops it rarely moves. The appendix may lie almost entirely in the pelvis, giving rise to tenderness only on rectal palpation. A retrocecal appendix may form an abscess yet produce no detectable signs of peritonitis. Localization by omentum may produce a mass found on abdominal or rectal palpation and may only be discovered after sedation or anesthesia has been induced.

On examination of the abdomen local tenderness, percussion tenderness, and local rebound tenderness are expected. As peritonitis develops, muscle guarding appears in the right lower quadrant and shortly in other quadrants. Remote tenderness and remote rebound tenderness appear as peritonitis spreads. A typical sequence of events may develop and local signs of peritonitis appear only to be followed by an unexpected relief of pain. This relief may be serious and should not interrupt treatment. Relief of pain may be caused by gangrene or perforation of the appendix rather than resolution. Recovery can be assumed only if relief of pain is gradual and is accompanied by lowering of fever, pulse, and leukocytosis and return of appetite.

There is no single diagnostic test for acute appendicitis. Because of the many variations, acute appendicitis must be considered in those patients having persisting lower abdominal pain. Appendicitis is uncommon in the first two years of life when spontaneous intussusception is most common. In the elderly the obstruction of colonic carcinoma may be as likely as appendicitis. In spite of the uncertainties careful attention to the sequence of visceral pain,

gastrointestinal upset, and right lower quadrant pain and signs of peritonitis and infection should lead the surgeon to remove no more than one normal appendix for every five acutely inflamed appendices. When the diagnosis of acute appendicitis is in doubt, observation in the hospital by a surgeon is safest.

Acute appendicitis during pregnancy is often difficult to diagnose and carries higher risk. As the pregnancy develops, the cecum and appendix rise higher in the abdomen shifting the usual right lower quadrant signs to higher levels. The patient's resistance and her response to infection may be reduced. Because the risk of acute peritonitis is greater in patients with acute appendicitis during pregnancy, early appendectomy is advisable.

When the symptoms and signs of acute appendicitis are present with gross abdominal distension, be aware of a possible second diagnosis. Right lower quadrant abdominal pain may be secondary to cecal distension that may be part of colonic distension proximal to an obstruction. If the obstruction is on the right side of the abdomen, the cecum and ascending colon are distended along with a section of small bowel. If the obstruction is on the left side of the abdomen or in the pelvis, plain X-rays reveal gaseous distension of the whole colon proximal to the obstruction. Acute appendicitis may be caused by granulomatous colitis of the cecum or a cecal carcinoma.

The types and distribution of pain from the appendix are:

Sensory innervation: Thoracic and lumbar splanchnic nerves (T10–L1) and vagus nerves (X), superior mesenteric plexus

Visceral pain: Umbilical

Somatic pain: Right lower quadrant at McBurney's point over the appendix

Referred pain: Rare

PROXIMAL COLON

The colon proximal to the splenic flexure develops from the midgut. Visceral pain from the proximal colon is felt in the midline in the periumbilical region. Periumbilical visceral pain caused by disease in the proximal colon cannot be distinguished from periumbilical visceral pain from diseases in other parts of the midgut. Balloon distension experiments and gaseous distension of the right colon during colonoscopy cause periumbilical visceral pain. With excessive distension of the ascending colon and cecum, right-sided abdominal pain may be felt. Right-sided pain caused by distension of the normal ascending colon or cecum is believed to be caused by traction on the parietal peritoneum since the ascending colon is fixed to the parietal peritoneum during development in the third stage of intestinal rotation. If fixation is incomplete, right-sided pain may not occur despite severe distension. An example of this is the periumbilical rather than the right-sided pain of nonstrangulated volvulus of the cecum. Gas seen by X-ray in the hepatic flexure of the unobstructed colon is an unlikely explanation for right-sided upper abdominal pain. Obstructions, inflammations, or infiltrating lesions of the ascending colon cause right-sided parietal pain by stimulating the parietal peritoneum. Similar lesions of the transverse colon are not associated with parietal pain so early, because the transverse colon has no direct attachment to the parietal peritoneum except at the hepatic and splenic flexures. Visceral pain from the transverse colon is felt in the umbilical region.

The types and distribution of pain from the ascending and transverse sections of the colon are summarized as follows:

Sensory innervation: Thoracic and lumbar splanchnic nerves (T10–L1) and vagus nerves (X), superior mesenteric plexus

Visceral pain: Umbilical, occasionally right flank from the ascending colon

Somatic pain: Over the site of the irritation

Referred pain: Rare

DISTAL COLON

The descending colon and sigmoid develop from the hindgut proximal to the cloaca. Visceral pain is felt in the midline in the suprapubic region unless the distension of the descending colon is severe. As on the right side of the abdomen, severe distension of the descending colon may cause left-sided abdominal pain by traction on the parietal peritoneum. Gaseous distension of the splenic flexure of the colon can cause left upper quadrant abdominal pain, but before that diagnosis is made a distal obstructing lesion of the colon must be eliminated with certainty. A serious error influencing the patient's survival can be made if the diagnosis of splenic flexure syndrome is accepted without complete examination of the distal colon.

The sigmoid colon is attached to the parietal peritoneum only at either end. Visceral pain caused by sigmoid colon distension is felt in the midline in the hypogastric region. The distension of the colon with sigmoid volvulus causes lower abdominal midline pain, but the severity of the pain varies with the rapidity of the distension. Slow distension of the sigmoid colon may be pain free. A sigmoid volvulus can be enormous without much pain.

Pain derived from the descending and sigmoid sections of the colon occurs at follows:

Sensory innervation: Thoracic and lumbar splanchnic nerves (T12–L1), inferior mesenteric plexus

Visceral pain: Hypogastrium, occasionally left flank from the descending colon

Somatic pain: Over the irritation
Referred pain: Rare

The colon and the rectum are the most common sites for carcinoma of the gastrointestinal tract. Unfortunately there is no discomfort associated with this growth until constipation, diarrhea, obstruction, or infiltration outside the bowel occurs. Be alert to investigate any recent change in bowel habits as this may be the only symptom of a curable colonic cancer.

Diverticulosis occurs most frequently and most extensively in the sigmoid colon; however, the bleeding it causes results in discomfort only when large amounts of blood in the colon stimulate peristalsis and evacuation. The only other complication of diverticulosis is acute diverticulitis, which is associated with pain and tenderness varying with the severity of the infection and the complications. Left lower quadrant abdominal pain and tenderness are not diagnostic of diverticulitis but diverticulitis is the most common cause of inflammation in the sigmoid colon.

The proximal hindgut is supplied by the inferior mesenteric artery. Slow occlusion of this artery is without effect. Rapid or sudden occlusion may produce ischemia of the descending and sigmoid portions of the colon especially if the marginal arteries at the splenic flexure and in the upper rectum are impaired. Narrowing of the inferior mesenteric artery with poor marginal circulation at either end of the proximal hindgut may cause hemorrhagic infarction. Ischemic infarction occurs if the arterial supply from all three directions stops. With sudden arterial occlusion sudden pain is felt and the bowel is stimulated to mass contraction and evacuation. Watery diarrhea occurs that may change to bloody diarrhea if hemorrhagic infarction occurs. Lesser degrees of ischemia may be recognized by barium X-ray, which shows swelling of the lining of the bowel caused by edema or hemorrhage in the submucosa. Congestion and edema are seen also on endoscopy (8). If gas is present in the sigmoid colon, thickening of the bowel wall may be recognized on supine plain films of the abdomen.

Spastic colon, mucous colitis, or irritable colon are names for the same syndrome. It has two pain patterns: either hypogastric and left lower abdominal cramps and often frequency and urgency of the bowels with small stools or steady abdominal discomfort, gaseous distension, and constipation. Treatment is symptomatic and for many patients unsatisfactory. Gas bloat syndrome and splenic flexure syndrome are related disorders. Stress often precipitates an attack. The etiology of these common syndromes is poorly understood.

RECTUM

The rectum develops from the cloaca, a derivative of the distal portion of the hindgut. The arterial supply of the cloaca is the internal iliac arteries. The main afferent nerve supply comes from the third and fourth sacral nerves. Visceral pain from the cloaca is felt centrally in the pelvis and is often referred posteriorly to the midsacral region. The pelvic peritoneum is supplied by these same sacral segments so that pelvic peritoneal irritation is also felt deep in the pelvis and often posteriorly in the midsacral region. Since there is no representation of sacral segments on the anterior abdominal wall, involuntary reflex contraction of abdominal wall muscles does not occur with severe visceral or parietal pain carried by the third or fourth sacral nerves. If the stimulant causing pelvic peritoneal irritation extends to the abdominal cavity, the abdominal pain, tenderness, and guarding of acute peritonitis appear. Types and distribution of pain from the rectum and upper anus are:

Sensory innervation: Pelvic splanchnic nerves (S3, 4) pelvic plexuses
Visceral pain: Central pelvis
Somatic pain: Central pelvis
Referred pain: Midsacral region in the midline

A variety of discomforts occur in the rectum, such as that of rapid distension. Inflammation and infiltration of the rectum produce deep pelvic pain and midsacral back pain. The pain caused by a growing neoplasm overfilling the pelvis is a terrible distress. Tenesmus, painful ineffectual straining at stool, may be caused by inflammation or infiltration of the rectum, prostate, cervix, or base of the urinary bladder. Proctalgia fugax is an intermittent and apparently severe pain in the rectum and anal canal thought to be spasmodic contraction of striated muscles in the pelvis or perineum. Solitary ulcer of the rectum is a rare lesion and the type of pain associated with it is difficult to understand. The lesion occurs in the rectal wall above the anal canal; yet the pain is burning and superficial. Burning pain is characteristic also of peptic ulcer disease in the duodenum or stomach. These burning pains are the only examples of superficial pain arising from viscera lined with glandular epithelium. The burning pain of reflux esophagitis and esophageal carcinoma and the burning of urinary cystitis occur in organs lined with other types of mucosa.

UTERUS, FALLOPIAN TUBES, AND OVARIES

The fallopian tubes and the body of the uterus have a similar nerve supply. The 12th thoracic and 1st lumbar nerves send afferent fibers through the lumbar sympathetic ganglia to the preaortic plexus and downward through the hypogastric plexus or presacral nerve, to the bilateral pelvic plexuses where sensory fibers join branches of the internal iliac arteries that pass to the uterus and tubes. Visceral pain is felt in the suprapubic region in the midline if from the uterus or tubes, occasionally slightly to the same side in the suprapubic region if from a tube. When visceral pain from the uterus is severe, it may occasionally radiate to the upper lumbar region but more commonly to the groins (L1). Severe pain from the uterus, such as labor contractions, may be felt in the inner thighs (L2). Crampy or intermittent pain from the pelvic organs may arise from uterine contractions or occasionally from torsions of the tubes or ovaries. Pain from the uterus and fallopian tubes occurs as follows:

Sensory innervation: Thoracic and lumbar splanchnic branches (T12, L1), hypogastric plexus
Visceral pain: Hypogastrium, groin
Somatic pain: Over the irritation
Referred pain: Groin, occasionally inner thigh

The cervix of the uterus is supplied by afferents from the third and fourth sacral nerves. If the cervix is dilated, visceral pain is felt deep in the pelvis and in the midsacral region in the back. Similarly, inflammatory and infiltrating lesions produce steady, deep pelvic pain and midsacral back pain. Cervical and upper vaginal pain is distributed as:

Sensory innervation: Pelvic splanchnic nerves (S3, 4), pelvic plexuses
Visceral pain: Central pelvis
Somatic pain: Central pelvis
Referred pain: Midsacral region in the midline

The ovaries develop high in the posterior abdominal wall at the level of the developing kidney and have an afferent nerve supply from the 10th and 11th thoracic nerves. The ovaries are sensitive to direct pressure on bimanual examination. This pain is felt deep in the pelvis at the site of the pressure and may be felt in the umbilical region; if severe, it is associated with nausea.

Pain resulting from bleeding with ovulation can occasionally be quite severe and associated with lower abdominal guarding and pelvic and rectal tenderness, but it subsides within 24 hours as a rule. It occurs two weeks before menstruation so that its relationship to the preceding menstrual period varies according to the length of the current menstrual cycle.

Functional or neoplastic cysts may rupture resulting in sudden onset of pain whose severity depends on the cyst size and the nature of its contents. Some gynecological causes of acute pelvic pain are ectopic pregnancy, incomplete abortion, acute salpingitis, and rupture or torsion of an ovarian lesion. Ruptured ectopic pregnancy and incomplete abortion are disorders of early pregnancy and are characterized by pain and vaginal bleeding. Ectopic pregnancies almost always occur in the fallopian tubes. The uterine end of the fallopian tube is narrow and pregnancy developing there is prone to early rupture and profuse hemorrhage into the peritoneal cavity. An ectopic pregnancy in the wider lateral end of the fallopian tube develops over a longer period of time. It may remain unruptured, and distension may cause unilateral visceral pain felt in the suprapubic region on the same side. Slow leakage of blood may occur from such an ectopic pregnancy causing intermittent suprapubic pain, vaginal bleeding, anemia, and a pelvic hematocele or hematoma.

Abdominal pain during pregnancy is a diagnostic challenge. One must be always mindful of the fact that the pregnant woman is not exempt from any nonobstetrical cause for abdominal pain. In addition, uterine rupture or *abruptio placentae* may complicate the pregnancy. Late in pregnancy right upper abdominal pain associated with toxemia may result from swelling of the liver and herald an impending convulsion.

Uncomplicated uterine fibroids cause pain only when large enough to exert pressure on adjacent organs; fibroids this large are easily palpated. Some fibroids, such as subserous fibroids undergoing torsion, submucous fibroids undergoing expulsion, and fibroids with red degeneration during pregnancy, may cause pain while still small and difficult to detect. If pain is caused by fibroids, it is pelvic, not abdominal, and in the back it is midsacral rather than lumbosacral.

URINARY BLADDER

The urinary bladder develops from the anterior portion of the cloaca. The arterial supply is the internal iliac arteries. The afferent nerve supply to the vault of the bladder is from T11-L2 segments. The nerve supply to the base of the bladder is the third and fourth sacral nerves. There is also a significant somatic supply from the third and fourth sacral segments through the pudendal nerves (22, 23).

The types and distribution of pain from the vault of the urinary bladder are:

Sensory innervation: Thoracic and lumbar splanchnic nerves (T11-L2), hypogastric plexus
Visceral pain: Hypogastrium
Somatic pain: Suprapubic region
Referred pain: Groins

Distension of the urinary bladder causes suprapubic pain. The bladder is covered on two surfaces by parietal peritoneum, and distension increases the tension of the local peritoneal covering. Pain associated with distension of the urinary bladder may also be felt in the back in the upper lumbar region. This pain is more likely to be the result of distension of the renal pelvis rather than referred pain. As with other organs slow distension can be pain free, whereas rapid distension is painful. The pain of overdistension is promptly relieved when the bladder is emptied. Urinary bladder pain may also be caused by inflammation and neoplastic infiltration.

BASE OF BLADDER, URETHRA, AND PROSTATE

The afferent nerve supply to the base of the urinary bladder, urethra, and prostate is the third and fourth sacral nerves. Somatic pain is carried by the pudendal nerves from the third and fourth sacral segments. Pain from these structures is felt deep in the pelvis and in the perineum. Pain may be referred to the midsacral region or to the urethral orifice. Inflammation of the base of the bladder or urethra produces a burning sensation felt most severely at the end of urination. Urgency, frequency, dysuria, and tenesmus are common.

The types and distribution of pain from these structures are as follows:

Sensory innervation: Pelvic splanchnic nerves (S3, 4) pelvic plexuses
Visceral pain: Central pelvis
Somatic pain: Central pelvis
Referred pain: (*a*) Midsacral region of the back, (*b*) distal end of the urethra

KIDNEY

The main visceral afferent supply of the kidney is the T10–L1 segments. The peripheral process passes through the splanchnic nerves, the white ramus communicans through the sympathetic ganglia, thoracic and lumbar sympathetic nerves to the preaortic plexus, and the renal plexus surrounding the renal arteries (35).

Pain and tenderness associated with kidney disease are felt in the angle between the 12th rib and the lateral border of the erector spinae muscles. It is often called the costovertebral angle although it is more accurate to call this the costomuscular angle. On very rare occasions pain arising from one kidney is felt in the costomuscular region on the opposite side of the body. Visceral pain from the kidney is rarely referred. Steady costomuscular pain may be caused by a calyceal stone or neoplasm.

Kidney and upper ureter pain occurs as:

Sensory innervation: Thoracic, least, and lumbar splanchnic nerves (T10–L1), renal plexus
Visceral pain: Costomuscular region
Somatic pain: Over the irritation
Referred pain: Rare

RENAL PELVIS AND URETER

The renal pelvis and upper ureter receive afferent nerves through the renal plexus from T10–L1 segments. Pain from the renal pelvis and upper end of the ureter is felt in the back in the costomuscular angle on the same side of the body. The pain caused by a ureteropelvic blockage is confined to the back. Obstruction of the lower ureter causes pain that is also felt in the costomuscular angle and may be referred to the groin and scrotum or labium on the same side (4). Pain from the lower ureter is found as follows:

Sensory innervation: Thoracic, least, and lumbar splanchnic nerves (T10–L1), renal plexus
Visceral pain: Costomuscular region, loin
Somatic pain: Lower abdominal quadrant over the irritation
Referred pain: Groin, scrotum, labia

Pain associated with kidney disease has many causes—injury, infection, or neoplastic infiltration arising from the kidney or renal pelvis. The most common cause of pain in the kidney is a distal urinary obstruction with distension of the renal pelvis. Again slow distension may be painless but rapid distension is painful. Slow distension results in hydronephrosis, commonly caused by a congenital abnormality at the ureteropelvic junction. The obstruction may be intermittent and recurrent. When pain is caused by intermittent ureteropelvic obstruction on the right side, it may be mistaken for biliary colic (12). Pain caused by distension of the ureter or renal pelvis is easily reproduced by retrograde pyelography under local anesthesia or by diuresis. Pain from the kidney is often associated with reflex paralytic ileus.

Sudden or rapid obstruction causes a steady distress resulting from the increasing distension of the renal pelvis. Renal colic is a steady continuous pain beginning insidiously, rapidly progressing to a plateau, and gradually subsiding unless aborted by narcotics. Renal colic is a severe pain lasting 10 minutes or longer and recurring no more frequently than every 30 minutes. Generally renal colic lasts 1-6 hours and occasionally up to 24 hours. It is unusual to have two attacks of renal colic in 24 hours. Although the summit may seem to fluctuate, the pain is constant and there is no relief during the attack. The patient remains in pain until the obstruction is relieved or narcotics are given. Renal colic resembles biliary colic. It is not like small bowel cramps, and the two should never be in the same differential diagnosis.

Patients often indicate the site of renal colic in the back by the back of their hand over the costomuscular angle, the palm of their hand on the loin, and their fingers on the inguinal region or groin. At times the pain is excruciating and causes the patient to squirm, roll about, and double up. The most common cause of ureteral obstruction is a stone. If the stone lodges in the lower ureter the pain is also felt in the lower abdomen or groin on the same side. It may be associated with urgent, frequent, and burning urination. There is evidence that the pain of ureteral colic is caused by distension rather than muscle contraction since the amplitude of contraction pressure remains within the normal range and falls as the ureter dilates (20).

TESTIS

The testis, like the ovary, arises from the embryonic tissues lying medial to the developing kidney and derives visceral innervation from the 10th and 11th segments. Pain from the testis is felt in the groin and lower abdomen on the same side (4). It is well known that the testis is sensitive to injury. Sudden injury produces severe visceral pain in the groin and lower abdomen and is associated with weakness, nausea, and vomiting. The tunica vaginalis is innervated by the genital branch of the genitofemoral nerve, and pain may be felt in the scrotum or groin. The scrotum is innervated by the pudendal nerve (S3, 4). A summary of the types and distribution of pain from the testis or ovary is:

Sensory innervation: Thoracic splanchnic nerves (T10, 11), renal plexus
Visceral pain: In the gonad
Somatic pain: Over the gonad
Referred pain: Umbilical region

ABDOMINAL AORTA AND ILIAC ARTERIES

Although dense plexuses of visceral afferent fibers lie on the anterior and lateral aspects of these vessels, pain arising from these vessels is rare except when they undergo enlargement or rupture. Slow narrowing by atherosclerosis with superimposed thrombosis causes lower limb fatigue, buttock claudication, symmetrical atrophy, pallor in the legs and feet, and inability to maintain erection of the penis. The main finding is absence of pulses in the lower limbs. The occlusion occurs below the renal vessels and is painless. Occlusion of an iliac artery is also painless if gradual; exercise causes claudication in the buttock and thigh. Sudden occlusion, however, is very painful producing pain at the level of the obstruction and distally in the limb. The effects of sudden arterial occlusion include pain, pallor, loss of distal pulses, loss of muscle power, and loss of skin sensation. The abdominal pain of aortic occlusion is usually overshadowed by pain in the lower back and thighs, shock, and paralysis.

The types and distribution of pain from the abdominal aorta are:

Sensory innervation: Lumbar nerves (L1-L4)
Somatic pain: Midline in the back opposite the upper four lumbar vertebrae
Referred pain: Rare

Aneurysm of the abdominal aorta may develop slowly and painlessly. Pain is associated with rapid enlargement, rupture, or dissection. As enlargement occurs the pain may range from vague lumbar, lumbosacral, and occasionally epigastric discomfort to severe pain. Excruciating back and flank pain suggests leakage or frank rupture of an aortic aneurysm, accompanied by signs of hypovolemic shock. Severe abdominal pain may mean premorbid intraperitoneal hemorrhage.

Physical examination usually reveals a pulsating abdominal mass at and above the umbilicus since most aneurysms of the abdominal aorta occur immediately below the renal vessels. The mass may be tender particularly if the aneurysm is expanding or leaking. There may be expansile or transmitted pulse or no pulse. The pulse in vessels distal to an abdominal aortic aneurysm should be palpable; extensive arteriosclerotic narrowing involving these vessels is quite rare. As a rule the lumen through an aortic aneurysm is patent; so there is no distal ischemia caused by the aneurysm. Dissecting aortic aneurysm is described below in the section on chest pain.

The following sections describe pain problems in nearby regions that may have to be considered in the differential diagnosis of abdominal pain.

BACK PAIN

As with pain in other regions, back pain demands a careful and complete history, full physical examination, and appropriate special investigations for diagnosis. The pain must be analyzed as to onset, location, radiation, quality, and aggravating and relieving factors. Back pain referred from disease in the abdomen or thorax should be recognized since careful functional inquiry uncovers symptoms of visceral disease. The careful examiner recognizes postural or structural abnormalities that may cause or aggravate back pain from other diseases. During interview and examination, psychogenic causative or aggravating factors are appreciated by the thoughtful physician.

Back pain caused by disease in the back means that some pain-sensitive structure is irritated. Periosteum, ligaments, fascia, muscles, sensory nerves, capsules of intervertebral joints, posterior roots and ganglia, and the spinal cord are the most sensitive structures in the back.

As a rule localized trauma is easily recognized from history and examination. Fracture of a bone as small as a lumbar transverse process may cause considerable local pain, tenderness, and painful limitation of motion. There is less protection and more flexibility in the cervical region than in the lumbar region so that fracture or dislocation is more common in the neck, but compression fracture occurs more often in the lumbar region.

Spondylolisthesis is a displacement of one part of the spine on another at a site of bone loss resulting from stress fracture or possibly a lack of fusion. The displacement causes strain on adjacent ligaments and joints; occasionally an entrapment of nerve roots occurs and causes sciatica. Protective muscle contraction increases the pain. A painful limitation of movement in the spine in that region is expected. Mild decalcification may be pain free, but more extensive osteoporosis causes widespread aching because of strain and loss of structural strength. More localized pain may occur with compression fracture or nerve root compression.

Infiltration by malignant growth in the spine causes constant pain intensified by weight bearing and movement. It is one of the few causes of back pain that is not relieved by rest and in fact frequently wakes the patient from sleep. As erosion occurs structural strength is lost and protective muscle spasm adds to the pain. Direct pressure, regional pounding, or sudden jarring increase the pain. Pain caused by malignant disease in bone has a steady, boring, expanding quality. It is severe, discouraging, and often poorly relieved by narcotics. Fortunately, it usually responds dramatically to radiation therapy.

Ankylosing spondylitis begins as a sacroiliac arthritis and spreads cranially involving intervertebral joints. Subligamentous calcification, protective spasm of muscles, irritation of nerve roots, and strain from stiffness make this a painful disease. The pain in the back eases as the spine fuses later in the disease. Nerve root irritation causes pain with sneezing, coughing, or other sudden movements that jar the spine. A patient with painful stiffness in the lumbar region should be investigated for this disease because earlier diagnosis leads to better treatment.

Osteoarthritis is a very common wear and tear degeneration that may occur in the spine. Irritation of fibrous tissues about the spine and degeneration of intervertebral joints cause the pain. The cartilage of the posterior intervertebral joints degenerates. Osteoarthritis occurs more frequently in the mobile lumbar and cervical regions of the spine. The pain is aching in character with sharp exacerbations on movement. Nerve root pressure may be another cause of pain. The lumbosacral joint suffers most often because of body weight, lordosis, and anterior tilting of the pelvis.

Herniated intervertebral disc is the most common cause of sciatica. Herniation often occurs suddenly while the patient is in a bent or stooped position. Irritation of the nerve root causes protective muscle spasm and lateral curvature of the spine; coughing and sneezing aggravate it. Spastic muscles become tender and painful. Although sciatic pain may be intermittent and aching, the pain tends to persist high in the midgluteal region. The pain of nerve root irritation is sharp and is associated with motor weakness, loss of reflexes, and dermatome hypoesthesia. Herniation of an intervertebral disc occurs most commonly in the lower segments of the lumbar and cervical regions of the spine.

Back strain or sprain results from incomplete tears or stretching of tendons, ligaments, or muscles so that pain and muscle spasm occur. The erector spinae, quadratus lumborum, latissimus dorsi, and trapezius muscles are most commonly affected. Muscle spasm may be secondary to painful lesions of the spinal column or primary when the muscle is directly irritated by myositis. Spastic muscles become painful and tender and stiffness develops. Fibrositis affects the back of the neck, shoulders, and scapular and lumbar regions. Acute fibrositis begins rapidly and produces intense spasm of regional muscles that may cause painful stiffness of the body and unusual attitudes and subsides fairly quickly. Chronic fibrositis is more insidious and is an aching rather than a painful condition. Stiffness is more evident after prolonged inactivity than while exercising. Improvement from chronic fibrositis is slow.

Lesions of the cord or meninges are not difficult to differentiate from musculoskeletal disorders as a rule. Trauma sufficient to cause damage to the spinal cord almost always causes fracture or dislocation of the spine. Meningeal irritation is shown by pain on neck flexion and painful neck stiffness related to sustained reflex contraction of back muscles in the neck region. Nerve root and nerve sheath irritation account for pain on straight leg raising and pain on extending the knee with the hip in flexion. By the time spinal cord tumors cause pain, usually there are sensory and motor changes on neurological examination.

Poor posture or structural abnormality may cause dull, aching, back pain, worse on standing, and relieved by sitting or lying. The pain comes from strains of muscles, tendon attachments, fascia, ligaments, and joint capsules. Structural abnormalities that cause such back pain include inequality of leg length, scoliosis, lordosis, kyphosis, but most commonly obesity. In the obese, loss of spinal flexibility, decreased tone of abdominal wall muscles, and the extra bulk supported by the spine are factors that increase the probability and severity of back pain.

It should be remembered that the most important extrinsic support for the lumbar spine is the anterior abdominal wall muscles. Poor tone of the abdominal wall muscles leads to certain backache. Patients who have back pain and have a laparotomy will have an increase in their back pain for three to six months following the laparotomy, until the abdominal wall strength returns to normal. Women who have backache have little change in the severity of the backache after vaginal hysterectomy, whereas after abdominal hysterectomy an increase in the severity and duration of the pain in the back is frequent.

Always remember that back pain may be caused by visceral disease. For example, peripheral lung lesions may irritate the posterior parietal pleura with regional pain in the back, shoulder, and sides before there is appreciable respiratory distress. Posterior mediastinal neoplasms may cause back pain. Aortic aneurysms cause back pain when they enlarge rapidly, leak, or dissect. As a rule abdominal disease causes abdominal pain before back pain. However, a liver or subphrenic abscess can cause shoulder-top pain before abdominal pain. Rarely back pain is the only pain felt in penetrating peptic ulcer (9). The back pain of penetrating peptic ulcer is felt at the same level in the back as the ulcer pain is felt in the epigastrium. Carcinoma of the pancreas may cause pain in the back only. A steady unrelenting back pain in the region of the first lumbar vertebra uninfluenced by posture or activity and without local tenderness demands investigation for carcinoma of the pancreas or other lesion in the upper abdomen.

The angle between the 12th rib and the lateral border of the erector spinae muscles is the typical site for the pain and tenderness of kidney disease. Steady pain in the midsacral region may be caused by disease in the sacrum or in pelvic structures derived from the cloaca in which case careful rectal and pelvic examination is likely to reveal the abnormality. Lumbosacral pain is more likely caused by a musculoskeletal disorder than abdominal visceral disease. Agonizing upper lumbar pain may be caused by acute pancreatitis, penetrating peptic ulcer, pancreatic neoplasm, aortic aneurysm, or local disease of the lumbar spine.

Certain features render the differentiation of visceral and musculoskeletal disorders difficult. When an inflammation or a painful infiltration is present, the pain is worse with movement and better with rest. Many painful visceral diseases are associated with reflex muscle spasm. As these muscles undergo sustained contraction, they become painful and tender. Occasionally trigger points occur that suggest rheumatic disease or fibrositis. A constant upper lumbar pain may suggest an inflammation or growth in the vertebral column, but it might be the earliest symptom of carcinoma of the body or tail of the pancreas. Pyelonephritis tends to cause constant back pain usually to one side at the angle between the 12th rib and the lateral border of the erector spinae muscles.

There are some features of value in differentiating painful musculoskeletal disease in the back from visceral disease with pain referred to the back. Musculoskeletal disease is greatly aggravated by movement and often completely relieved by rest. The limitation of movement is much greater with musculoskeletal disorders, and the amount of muscle spasm is greater than the spasm associated with visceral diseases. Tenderness in musculoskeletal disorders is well localized to the site. The movement allowed at painful joints is limited by sustained contraction of muscles that span the joint. By limiting movement, muscle contraction limits pain; the pain caused by attempted movement is worse than the pain from sustained muscle contraction alone. Musculoskeletal disease does not cause upset of visceral function; so there should be no common symptom of gastrointestinal disease such as anorexia, nausea, vomiting, cramps, or diarrhea. Musculoskeletal diseases and their neurological complications tend to be strictly segmental with sensory, motor, and reflex changes anatomically appropriate for the lesion.

LATERAL AND ANTERIOR ABDOMINAL WALLS

Abrupt onset of severe pain localized to one quadrant of the abdomen, usually the right or left lower, may be caused by hemorrhage into the rectus sheath. As a result the hematoma produces a firm immobile mass localized to a rectus muscle. It is as easily felt when the muscles are contracted as when they are relaxed. It tends to occur after strenuous effort (27) or in patients on anticoagulant therapy (13). It is rare.

Abdominal wall hernias, which are painful, are easily recognized because of the mass, the site, and the tenderness. The symptoms are intermittent when the hernia is reducible. When the hernia becomes irreducible, there is a constant mass, pain, tenderness, and the threat of strangulation. Diagnostic difficulties arise when a hernia is very small or at an unusual site. A very small paraumbilical hernia may produce symptoms by causing strangulation of a small tag of omentum or vague intra-abdominal symptoms probably caused by drag on the omentum. An epigastric hernia may cause vague upper abdominal symptoms that are confusing until the hernia is identified. Local anesthetic injection of the herniated extraperitoneal fat relieves the symptoms caused by this midline hernia.

Spigelian hernias occur most commonly at the lower lateral border of the posterior rectus sheath. Lumbar hernias rarely strangulate. When bowel obstruction occurs, the site of tenderness and the pattern of referred pain in the thigh might lead an astute surgeon to the correct preoperative diagnosis of a strangulated gluteal, sciatic, or obturator hernia. Each is very rare.

There are two lesions of posterior roots and posterior root ganglia that are caused by infection and may cause abdominal wall pain, herpes zoster and tabes dorsalis. Herpes zoster is caused by reactivation of a previous chickenpox virus infection in a posterior root ganglion. Reactivation of the viral infection may be spontaneous or the result of trauma, neoplasm, corticosteroid therapy, or immunosuppressive drugs (33). Pain appears in one or several adjacent dermatomes on one side of the body, three or four days before the appearance of the typical vesicular eruption. Pain creates diagnostic difficulty if it occurs before the rash. Control of the pain may be a major clinical problem. A syphilitic infection may be followed by tabes dorsalis 5 to 20 years later. Posterior root ganglion cells and their axons and myelin sheaths in the posterior columns of the cord undergo degeneration causing extensive neurological deficits. Paroxysmal pain may be a distressing symptom. These lightninglike pains resemble a series of knife stabs lasting a few moments or a few minutes and then shifting to another region. Sensory ataxia may include loss of visceral sensation. Tabetic crises may be characterized by acute epigastric pain, severe hyperesthesia, tenesmus, strangury, and faintness. Characteristic neurological deficits and appropriate examination of the serum and the cerebrospinal fluid make the diagnosis. Tabes dorsalis has become very rare.

Pain and tenderness may develop in the normally insensitive xiphoid process. It may become less flexible and may calcify. The lower end may bend forward producing a tender lump (25). Infiltration with local anesthetic agent proves the source of the pain, relieves patient worry, and permits physician reassurance.

CHEST WALL

Many conditions that affect the anterior and lateral abdominal walls also affect the thoracic walls. It is especially important to recognize pain arising from the chest walls because many of these patients will have assumed that they have serious heart disease. Often such explanation results in dramatic relief. Painful conditions of the thoracic walls are common; very few are serious. The alcoholic may not be able to recall the injury that caused rib fracture. An enlarging aortic aneurysm may erode the chest wall and cause unremitting pain. New growths, particularly multiple myeloma, leukemia, and sarcoma, may invade ribs. Metastatic carcinoma from breast and prostate and hypernephroma commonly involve ribs. Tuberculous or other infections of the ribs may be responsible for pain. In most of these conditions there is a point of tenderness at the site of pain and a fusiform mass may be found. X-ray examination and radioisotope scans of the ribs may be needed.

Rib cartilages tend to remain painful much longer after trauma than rib fractures. The costochondral junction is prone to prolonged pain and tenderness following injury. Slipping rib cartilages are a frequent cause of chest pain (15). Ribs also may slip one upon another and in either case patients may notice a painful click. The lower five or six ribs and cartilages are most often affected. Relief of pain following local anesthetic infiltration demonstrates the nature of the problem to the worried patient. Inflammation of the upper costal cartilages, Tietze's syndrome, is characterized by aching pain, tenderness in the cartilage, and sometimes a fusiform swelling of the cartilage. Anti-inflammatory drugs provide gradual relief (19).

Toxic or inflammatory irritation of posterior nerve roots causes pain at the point of irritation and pain referred in the peripheral distribution of the nerve. Local pressure from an extruded lower cervical intervertebral disc, swelling of an intervertebral joint, tabes dorsalis, or herpes zoster may cause nerve root pain. Thoracic deformity alone may cause intercostal nerve pain. Spinal nerve root pain is often mistaken for cardiac pain (7).

The muscles of the thoracic girdle and neck are frequent sites for fibrositis and fibromyositis. Almost everyone has experienced aching pain in these muscles after unusual effort, especially when their physical condition is poor. Aching muscles are tender. Muscle spasms or cramps occur in the intercostal muscles similar to the painful cramps that occur in leg muscles. Young, healthy adults may have a precordial catch or spasm with momentary sharp, localized pain increased by inspiration and immediately abolished by bending and stretching (24). Whenever chest pain lasts only one or two seconds, complete reassurance can be given the patient. Bornholm disease is an epidemic myalgia or pleurodynia caused by the Coxsackie B virus. This disease causes episodes of pain in the chest and abdomen and appears to involve the diaphragm and intercostal and abdominal wall muscles. The diagnosis of the condition is difficult when it occurs sporadically.

Mondor's disease is an acute phlebitis of unknown cause in a superficial chest wall vein. A cervical rib can cause a compression syndrome with shoulder and arm pain that may be confused with intrathoracic disease. Careful history and physical examination and awareness of chest wall conditions generally lead to the correct diagnosis and allow the physician to give positive and complete reassurance that such pain is not caused by serious heart disease.

TRACHEA, BRONCHI, AND LUNGS

The trachea is sensitive to most of the stimuli that produce superficial pain in the skin. Inflammation resulting from injury caused by inhalation of irritating gases, foreign bodies, or infection increases the sensitivity of the tracheal mucosa to pain. The pain is well localized to the upper sternal region at the level of the irritation. The large bronchi have similar sensibility and stimulation of the mucosa of a bronchus causes pain on the same side. The pain appears to be carried exclusively in the vagus nerves (30). The pain of acute tracheitis is burning in nature and felt deep to the upper sternum. It is accentuated by coughing.

The small bronchi, bronchioles, lung parenchyma, and visceral pleura are insensitive. All pain arising from pleura depends upon irritation of the parietal pleura. The sensitivity of the parietal pleura and the complete insensitivity of the visceral pleura and lung are readily demonstrated during thoracoscopy under local anesthesia. Parietal pleural irritation results in sharply localized, clear, intense pain accentuated by any respiratory movement. Laughing, coughing, or regular breathing causes pain, whereas holding the breath avoids it. The periphery of the diaphragm is innervated by the lower six intercostal nerves. The central portion of the diaphragm is innervated by the phrenic nerve from the third, fourth, and fifth cervical spinal nerves. Pain from stimulation of the peripheral part of the diaphragm is felt on the same side over the adjacent lower ribs. Pain from the central portion of the diaphragm is felt on the top of the shoulder near the anterior border of the trapezius muscle on the same side (5).

A sizable pulmonary infarct causes sudden, unilateral pleuritic chest pain, shortness of breath, hemoptysis, cyanosis, and fear. The wheezing of bronchospasm may be a prominent symptom. A massive pulmonary embolus may cause pain resembling myocardial infarction. Typical candidates for pulmonary embolus include pregnant women; women taking oral contraceptives; inactive obese individuals; and patients recovering from myocardial infarction, cerebral thrombosis, surgical operation, or extensive injury. The source of the embolus may be suggested by obvious thrombophlebitis, swelling of one calf, calf tenderness, or Homan's sign. Chest X-ray may show the infarct or its effects. Dyspnea, apprehension, unexplained sinus tachycardia, elevated jugular venous pressure, accentuated second pulmonic sound, and right ventricular gallop rhythm suggest pulmonary embolus. An electrocardiogram may indicate pulmonary embolism especially if previous electrocardiograms are available for comparison. Small emboli may precede a massive embolus by several hours or days. Early recognition and treatment of multiple small emboli may prevent fatal pulmonary embolism.

Slow onset pneumothorax may be pain free, but rapid onset pneumothorax causes sudden sharp chest pain in the shoulder and back on the same side. The pain may be caused by sudden pull on the parietal pleura by pleural adhesions (26). Dyspnea, orthopnea, anxiety, and pain on deep inspiration are expected. Clinical and radiological signs of pneumothorax are easily found.

Pleurisy or acute pleuritis produces unilateral chest pain that is unusually sharp, aggravated by inspiration, and frequently associated with cough and dyspnea. The pain is relieved when the breath is held. Pleuritic pain and a friction rub usually disappear as a pleural effusion develops. Although pleurisy is easy to identify, it is usually a complication of underlying lung disease, which may be difficult to diagnose.

It is tragic that bronchogenic carcinoma is pain free until spread or complications occur. The complications of atelectasis, pneumonitis, and abscess produce pain. Invasion of pleura, ribs, and brachial plexus cause local pain (32), whereas metastases in distant structures, especially bones, cause remote pain. Pain may precede paralysis or anesthesia as the tumor invades the recurrent laryngeal or phrenic nerves, the cervical and thoracic sympathetic nerves and ganglia, and somatic branches of cervical and thoracic spinal nerves.

CARDIAC PAIN

Heart pain, other than pericardial pain, appears to come almost entirely from the myocardium. The prime cause of pain from the myocardium is ischemia, which causes pain by hypoxia of the muscle with accumulation of metabolites. The usual physical cause of myocardial ischemia is arteriosclerotic narrowing of the coronary arteries. There may be an absolute diminution in coronary blood flow or an increased demand on the heart pushing it beyond its available blood supply as may happen with ventricular hypertrophy or heart valve disease.

Sensory fibers to the myocardium have their cell bodies in the dorsal root ganglia of the upper six thoracic nerves (3). The peripheral processes run through the spinal nerves, white rami, sympathetic trunk, the upper six thoracic and the two or three cervical sympathetic ganglia, and splanchnic branches to the cardiac plexus, reaching the myocardium by the periarterial plexuses of the coronary arteries (41). Other branches of the upper six thoracic nerves spread to the whole of the upper half of the body except the scalp. It is easy to appreciate how cranial spread of severe pain from the myocardium can be felt in the chest, arms, neck, and face. Types and distribution of pain from the heart are:

Sensory innervation: Cervical and thoracic splanchnic branches (T1–6) and vagus nerves (X), cardiac plexus

Visceral pain: Central chest

Somatic pain: Central chest

Referred pain: (*a*) Shoulders and arms especially on the left side, (*b*) neck and jaws, (*c*) upper thoracic region in the back, (*d*) epigastrium

During development the straight heart tube folds and begins to separate into two before sensory fibers penetrate the myocardium. Bilateral innervation accounts for the midline retrosternal location of typical myocardial pain. Severe myocardial ischemia occurs more frequently in the walls of the left ventricle, and this probably accounts for the more frequent radiation of pain to the left shoulder and the left inner arm and back. Nerve fibers passing through the cervical sympathetic ganglia are distributed widely in the periarterial plexuses of the branches of the external carotid vessels; they account for the spread of severe myocardial pain to the jaws, throat, tongue, palate, and pharynx (3). When myocardial pain is severe, spread of pain is extensive and reflex contraction of the regional muscles occurs. The symptoms of substernal oppression are caused by reflex sustained contraction of intercostal muscles (26). Similarly severe visceral pain from the myocardium is associated with reflex autonomic phenomena such as sweating, ashen cyanosis, lowered blood pressure, weakened pulse, nausea, and vomiting. The psychic reaction to severe visceral pain, particularly where there is suspicion of heart disease, is prominent. Some of the spinal segments supplying the heart with sensory fibers also supply the esophagus and the foregut. Angina pectoris, diffuse esophageal spasm, and biliary colic are often problems in differential diagnosis.

Chest pain from myocardial ischemia presents a spectrum of entities from mild angina pectoris, through acute coronary insufficiency, to extensive myocardial infarction. The quality of these pains is similar; the main differences are the duration and severity of the pain and the aggravating and relieving factors.

Angina Pectoris

Angina pectoris is characterized by attacks of pain or oppression situated in the midline retrosternally, precipitated by activity and other factors, and relieved by rest and nitroglycerin. The character of the distress may be identified by the patient as a discomfort rather than a pain. The distress or discomfort may be described as squeezing, pressing, suffocating, tightening, constricting, expanding, burning, numbing, viselike, breaking, or as a heaviness or indigestion. The sensation is easy to identify when typical, but there are many exceptions. The pain may be superficial and felt off the midline, in the shoulder, arms, hands, neck, jaws, throat, cheeks, mastoids, or epigastrium.

It must be realized that substernal pain radiating to the left arm is frequently encountered in patients with functional or other noncardiac disorders (24). As a rule the more severe the discomfort, the more widely it radiates. There may be pain in the epigastrium or other remote area and no pain in the chest. The severity of cardiac pain does not necessarily indicate its gravity. The usual precipitating causes are effort, emotion, intercourse, meals, and cold weather. When angina pectoris is induced by exertion, it as a rule begins mildly and becomes progressively more severe until the patient is forced to rest. A second effort may be possible to a much greater degree without any distress whatsoever, a second wind effect. Anginal pain starting at rest or during the night, nocturnal angina, usually indicates a more advanced and unstable degree of myocardial ischemia. Excitement may cause angina pectoris in a patient capable of moderate activity without distress. When angina pectoris occurs, many patients become anxious and this increases their distress. Tachycardia may be the link between excitement and angina. The extra myocardial effort brought on by increased splanchnic blood flow after meals can precipitate angina pectoris. The supine position with improved venous return from the legs places further effort on the heart so that after meals angina patients should rest in the sitting rather than in the supine position.

Angina pectoris may be precipitated by cold. This is thought to be caused by an increase in peripheral resistance that increases myocardial work and oxygen consumption. Often several of these typical precipitating factors can be blamed for an attack of angina pectoris. An ideal set of conditions for precipitating an attack would be represented by a man climbing a hill against a cold wind, carrying a suitcase, having just eaten, and engaging in a heated conversation (26). Angina pectoris is a possibility in all adult men; it is unusual in premenopausal women unless they are diabetic or hypertensive.

When activity is the dominant precipitating cause for angina pectoris, relief from the pain occurs after a short period of rest. If pain suspected of myocardial ischemia lasts less than $\frac{1}{2}$ minute, the diagnosis of angina pectoris is in serious doubt; if longer than 20 minutes, suspect coronary insufficiency or myocardial infarction. The pain of angina pectoris should be relieved within 3 minutes by sublingual nitroglycerin. If relief comes after 5 minutes, the diagnosis is in doubt, and pain relief after 10 minutes is not the result of the nitroglycerin. Failure to respond to nitroglycerin does not exclude coronary insufficiency. The potency and absorption of nitroglycerin are demonstrated by a feeling of flushing in the face and throbbing in the head. Biliary colic and esophageal spasm may be improved by nitroglycerin but not within the first minute or two. Nitroglycerin provides a useful diagnostic test. A test considered dangerous is the induction of sinus bradycardia by carotid sinus massage, which relieves angina but not noncardiac pain (23).

Physical examination may be of little help in diagnosis. Abnormal physical findings may be present in patients having noncardiac pain. The physical abnormalities in patients with angina may include an S4 gallop, transient murmur of mitral insufficiency, and arrhythmias. The resting electrocardiogram is often normal; nonspecific abnormalities in the electrocardiogram should not be taken as proof that the patient with unusual chest pain has myocardial ischemia. When there are atypical features the electrocardiographic response to exercise may be used provided there are no contraindications.

Acute Coronary Insufficiency

Acute coronary insufficiency is prolonged angina pectoris pain caused by myocardial ischemia but not followed by the electrocardiographic or enzyme changes of myocardial infarction. The pain lasts more than 20 minutes with incomplete or no relief with coronary vasodilators. As a rule there is no precipitating cause, but occasionally one may identify tachycardia, anemia, or thyrotoxicosis. The pain may last for several hours and is not relieved by rest. An electrocardiogram may be normal when there is no pain but a normal electrocardiogram during an attack of pain is evidence, although not conclusive, against myocardial ischemia. The transient electrocardiographic changes are those of ischemia but not of infarction.

Crescendo angina refers to the increasing frequency of attacks of angina, duration of less than 15 minutes, and prompt relief with a coronary vasodilator. Recurring attacks of acute coronary insufficiency or crescendo angina may precede myocardial infarction. Patients having crescendo angina or acute coronary insufficiency deserve prompt medical care and investigation for aortocoronary bypass.

Acute Myocardial Infarction

Acute myocardial infarction produces the same kind of pain with the same distribution as both angina pectoris and acute coronary insufficiency. The pain is usually more severe, more difficult to control, and may last several hours. It rarely begins suddenly but attains its peak of severity quickly. In many cases over a period of days or weeks there may have been recurring mild chest discomfort or indigestion often following some unusual stress or effort, that is, preinfarction angina. There may be a past history of coronary artery disease.

Sweating, tachycardia, and dyspnea occur in each of the three types of myocardial ischemic pain but are most evident in cases of infarction. Clinical evidence of shock with falling blood pressure does not occur in angina pectoris and rarely in acute coronary insufficiency. Fever, leukocytosis, and pericardial friction rub occur only with myocardial infarction. At first the electrocardiogram may be normal, but soon it and the concentration of appropriate serum enzymes become diagnostic. Failure to recognize serious coronary artery disease is dangerous and a threat to the patient's survival. On the other hand the incorrect diagnosis of serious heart disease can lead to prolonged cardiac invalidism, an incapacity that is very difficult to reverse. Every patient in pain suffers more when the physician is uncertain or when there are conflicting opinions.

Mitral Click Syndrome (Mitral Valve Prolapse)

This syndrome is very common particularly in young women. There may be myxomatous degeneration of one or both mitral leaflets and chordae tendinae leading to redundancy of valve tissue and prolapse into the left atrium during systole. With maximum prolapse there is a nonejection click. Mitral regurgitation, while usually absent or minimal, may become severe because of ruptured chordae or bacterial endocarditis. Chest pain and cardiac arrhythmias are outstanding features and the electrocardiogram may show nonspecific T-wave abnormality. It is important to recognize this condition as it is generally innocent.

Pericardial Pain

Experimental stimulation under local anesthesia shows that the visceral pericardium is insensitive, but the lower parietal pericardium is sensitive to scratch (5). The pain of pericarditis is often severe and sudden in onset. It is clear, sharp, and increases with inspiration and motion of the trunk. Leaning forward appears to afford some relief. This pain may be partly caused by an associated pleurisy and may be felt in the epigastrium. Swallowing or coughing may aggravate pericardial pain. Rarely the pain is intermittent and coincident with the pulse. Idiopathic or viral pericarditis may follow an upper respiratory infection.

Acute pericarditis is most apt to be confused with acute myocardial infarction. If the patient has been under observation from the onset of the pain, the differentiation may not be difficult. Chest pain, fever, leukocytosis, and pericardial friction rub are present from the onset of acute pericarditis, whereas fever, leukocytosis, and pericardial friction rub may appear only 24–48 hours after the onset of the pain in myocardial infarction. As a pericardial effusion develops the friction rub may disappear. Confirmatory evidence may be obtained from the electrocardiogram, especially if serial recordings are available.

PAIN FROM THE AORTA

Pain from disease of the aorta may be sudden and severe. Early recognition is needed for early successful treatment. Disease of the aorta must be kept in mind when sudden onset of severe chest pain occurs in patients who are hypertensive, pregnant, injured, or who have coarctation or Marfan's syndrome (24).

Dissecting aneurysm of the aorta is a complication of cystic medial necrosis (37). An intimal tear leads to hematoma in the media, splitting the aorta. Excruciating interscapular back pain first suggests that the dissection begins in the distal arch of the aorta just beyond the left subclavian artery. The pain is most severe at the onset. The tearing pain caused by the dissection spreads downwards; it is probably related to the moving origin of the pain. There may be vasoconstriction of distal vessels, especially in the lower extremities, similar to an acute occlusion of the abdominal aorta with loss of pulses, paralysis, pain, and pallor.

There may be an aortic insufficiency murmur if the root of the aorta is involved and diminished heart sounds if cardiac tamponade has occurred. Urinary flow decreases and bizarre neurological deficits occur as the blood supply to the cord decreases. Most patients are hypertensive and pharmacological reduction of the blood pressure slows the dissection and reduces the pain. The electrocardiogram may be normal or may rarely show myocardial infarction if coronary arteries are involved. X-rays may show widening of the mediastinum, left hemothorax, or a wide aorta; the aneurysm may be demonstrated by angiography. Pain relief on reducing the blood pressure by drugs may be used as a test to confirm the diagnosis. Chronic dissection is uncommon and less painful.

Eventually the very dilated aorta may cause boring retrosternal chest pain partly relieved by assuming a position that relieves pressure by the aneurysm on the thoracic cage. Sharp stabbing pain may be caused by pressure of the dilated aorta on pain-sensitive regional nerves.

Often an aortic aneurysm is found to be clotted and has no expansile pulse. In this case there may be a transmitted pulse as a lumen persists. The distal circulation is unimpaired. A pulsating or nonpulsating posterior mediastinal or retroperitoneal mass may be confused with neoplasm. Plain X-rays may show calcification in the widened aortic wall. Aortography is rarely needed.

CHEST PAIN OF GASTROINTESTINAL ORIGIN

Visceral pain from the myocardium and nonvisceral pain in the chest are often confused with pain arising from the gastrointestinal tract. Approximately one of four patients admitted to the hospital with precordial chest pain will be found to have a gastrointestinal disorder (2). About one of five patients referred for surgical treatment of biliary colic and gallstones has been examined by a cardiologist to rule out myocardial ischemia. Reflux esophagitis and hiatus hernia are the most common gastrointestinal abnormalities simulating myocardial ischemia (24). Chest pain resembling angina pectoris is the chief complaint of 5% of patients with hiatus hernia (31).

Esophageal pain is more commonly brought on by food than cardiac pain. It is usually a superficial pain of burning character promptly relieved on swallowing a liquid antacid if the pain is caused by reflux. Reflux is frequently brought on by lying down especially after taking a large meal or alcohol and relieved by sitting or standing. Burning pain on swallowing may arise from the lower esophagus in the presence of reflux esophagitis or may occur in the esophagus at any level because of carcinoma. Burning pain associated with a carcinoma is not significantly relieved by antacids, and careful questioning reveals increasing difficulty with swallowing.

Biliary colic may produce high epigastric or low retrosternal visceral midline pain resembling the pain of myocardial ischemia. Biliary colic usually lasts longer than 15 or 20 minutes and infrequently recurs within 24 hours. It is more likely to be confused with preinfarction angina than with stable angina pectoris. Increasing frequency of attacks might suggest crescendo angina. The location of the pain in the gallbladder region with local tenderness and radiation of pain to the inferior angle of the right scapula make the diagnosis of acute cholecystitis reasonably clear.

A large number of other gastrointestinal tract symptoms can be confused with the pain of myocardial ischemia. In most instances a careful analysis of the pain on thorough history taking followed by physical examination leads to the correct diagnosis. Sometimes the diagnosis is confirmed by a specific laboratory test. When the clinical picture is inconclusive or confusing and there is no specific test, all of the evidence is gathered and weighed and the most probable diagnosis chosen for further investigation or treatment. The ability to act on incomplete evidence is called the art of medicine.

REFERENCES

1. Beaumont W: Experiments and Observations on the Gastric Juice and the Physiology of Digestion, 1833. Facsimile of the original edition, XIII International Physiological Congress, Boston, 1929.
2. Bennett JR, Atkinson M: The differentiation between esophageal and cardiac pain. Lancet 2:1123–1127, 1966.

3. Bingham JR, Ingelfinger FJ, Smithwick RH: The effects of sympathectomy on abdominal pain in man. Gastroenterology 15:18–31, 1950.
4. Brown FR: Testicular pain. Lancet 1:994–999, 1949.
5. Capps JA, Coleman GH: An Experimental and Clinical Study of Pain in the Pleura, Pericardium and Peritoneum. New York: MacMillan, 1932.
6. Charney KJ, Juler GL, Comarr AE:General surgery problems in patients with spinal cord injuries. Arch Surg 110:1083–1088, 1975.
7. Davis D: Spinal nerve root pain (radiculitis) simulating coronary occlusion; a common syndrome. Am Heart J 35:70–80, 1948.
8. Ernest CA, Hagihara PF, Daugherty ME, Sachatello CR, Griffen Jr WO: Ischemic colitis incidence following abdominal aorta reconstruction: A prospective study. Surgery 80:417–421, 1976.
9. Gilson SB: Back pain in peptic ulcer. NY State J Med 61:625–626, 1961.
10. Greenfield J: Abdominal operations on patients with chronic paraplegia. Arch Surg 59:1077–1087, 1949.
11. Guyton AC: Textbook of Medical Physiology, 4th ed. Philadelphia: Saunders, 1971.
12. Halasz NA: Counterfeit cholecystitis. Am J Surg 130:189–193, 1975.
13. Hildreth DH: Anticoagulant therapy and rectus sheath hematoma. Am J Surg 124:80–86, 1972.
14. Hoen TI, Cooper IS: Acute abdominal emergencies in paraplegics. Am J Surg 75:19–24, 1948.
15. Holmes JF: Slipping rib cartilage with report of cases. Am J Surg 54:326–338, 1941.
16. Ingberg HO, Prust FW: The diagnosis of abdominal emergencies in patients with spinal cord lesions. Arch Phys Med 49:343–348, 1968.
17. Jones CM: Digestive Tract Pain: Diagnosis and Treatment Experimental Observations. New York: MacMillan, 1938.
18. Jones CM: Pain from the digestive tract. In: Pain, Proceedings of the Association for Research in Nervous and Mental Disease, Dec. 18–19, 1942, New York. pp. 274–288. Baltimore: Williams & Wilkins, 1943.
19. Kayser HL: Tietze's syndrome—A review of the literature. Am J Med 21:982–989, 1956.
20. Kiil F: Physiology of the renal pelvis and ureter. In: Urology, edited by MF Campbell, pp. 81–117. Philadelphia: Saunders, 1963.
21. Kingsnorth AN: Fluid filled intestinal obstruction. Br J Surg 63:289–291, 1976.
22. Learmonth JR: Neurosurgery in the treatment of disease of the urinary bladder. J Urol 26:13–24, 1931.
23. Levine SA: Carotid sinus massage. A new diagnostic test for angina pectoris. JAMA 182:1332–1334, 1962.
24. Lichstein E, Seckler SG: Evaluation of acute chest pain. Med Clin North Amer 57:1481–1490, 1973.
25. Lipkin ML, Fulton A, Wolfson EA: The syndrome of the hypersensitive xiphoid. N Engl J Med 253:591–597, 1955.
26. MacBryde CM: Signs and Symptoms, 5th ed. Philadelphia: Lippincott, 1970.

27. Manier JW: Rectus sheath hematoma. Am J Gastroenterol 7:443–452, 1972.
28. Marston A, Kieny R, Szilagyi E, Taylor GW: Intestinal ischemia. Arch Surg 111:107–112, 1976.
29. Mitchell GAG: Anatomy of the Autonomic Nervous System. Edinburgh: Livingstone, 1953.
30. Morton DR, Klassen KP, Curtis GM: The effect of high vagus section upon the clinical physiology of the bronchi. J Lab Clin Med 34:1730, 1949.
31. Palmer ED: Serious heart disease simulated by hiatus hernia. US Armed Forces Med J 8:477–480, 1957.
32. Pancoast HK: Superior pulmonary sulcus tumor. JAMA 99:1391–1396, 1932.
33. Passmore R, Robson JS: A Companion to Medical Studies. Oxford: Blackwell, 1974.
34. Polland WS, Bloomfield AD: Experimental referred pain from the gastrointestinal tract. J Clin Invest 10:435–452, 1931.
35. Ray BS, Neil CL: Abdominal visceral pain in man. Ann Surg 126:709–724, 1947.
36. Ruch TC, Patton HD: Physiology and Biophysics, 19th ed. Philadelphia: Saunders, 1965.
37. Sailer S: Dissecting aneurysm of the aorta. Arch Path 33:704–730, 1942.
38. Sullivan JA: Vascular disease of the intestines. Med Clin North Am 58:1473–1485, 1974.
39. White JC: Diagnostic novacaine block of the sensory and sympathetic nerves. Am J Surg 9:264–277, 1930.
40. White JC: Sensory Innervation of the Viscera. In: Pain, Proceedings of the Association for Research in Nervous and Mental Disease, Dec. 18–19, 1942, New York, pp. 373–390. Baltimore: Williams & Wilkins, 1943.
41. White JC: Cardiac pain: Anatomic pathways and physiologic mechanisms. Circ Res 5:644–655, 1957.
42. White TT, Lawinski M, Strachen G: Treatment of pancreatitis by left splanchnicectomy and celiac ganglionectomy. Am J Surg 112:195–196, 1966.
43. White JC, Smithwick RH, Simeone FA: The Autonomic Nervous System. New York: MacMillan, 1952.
44. White JC, Sweet WH: Pain and the Neurosurgeon. Springfield, Ill.: Thomas, 1969.
45. Wolff HG, Wolf S: Pain, 2d ed. Springfield, Ill.: Thomas, 1958.
46. Wolf S, Wolff HG: Human Gastric Function—An Experimental Study of a Man and His Stomach. London: Oxford, 1943.

FURTHER READING

Bretland PM: Acute Ureteric Obstruction. London: Butterworth, 1972.

Botsford TW, Wilson RE: The Acute Abdomen, 2d ed. Philadelphia: Saunders, 1977.

Cope Z: The Early Diagnosis of the Acute Abdomen, 14th ed. London: Oxford, 1972.

Dunphy JE, Way LW: Current Surgical Diagnosis and Treatment. Los Altos, Calif.: Lange, 1973.

Farmer DA: Abdominal pain. Med Clin North Am 41:1287–1302, 1957.

Gelin LE, Nyhus LM, Condon RE: Abdominal Pain. Philadelphia: Lippincott, 1969.

Hannington-Kiff JG: Pain Relief. Philadelphia: Lippincott, 1974.

Harvey AM, Bordley J: Differential Diagnosis, 2d ed. Philadelphia: Saunders, 1972.

Jones PF: Emergency Abdominal Surgery in Infancy, Childhood and Adult Life. Oxford: Blackwell, 1974.

Levene DL: Chest Pain: An Integrated Diagnostic Approach. Philadelphia: Lea & Febiger, 1977.

Lowenfels AB: Companion Guide to Surgical Diagnosis. Baltimore: Williams & Wilkins, 1975.

McMasters RE: A clinical approach to pain. South Med J 67:173–176, 1974.

McNab I: Backache. Philadelphia: Williams & Wilkins, 1977.

Mellinkoff SM: The Differential Diagnosis of Abdominal Pain. New York: McGraw-Hill, 1957.

Shepherd JA: A Concise Surgery of the Acute Abdomen. Edinburgh: Churchill, Livingstone, 1975.

Smithells RW: Medical conditions simulating the acute abdomen. Ann R Coll Surg Engl 48:23, 1971.

Steinheber FU: Medical conditions mimicking the acute surgical abdomen. Med Clin North Am 57:1559–1567, 1973.

Chapter 8

Diagnosis by Pattern Recognition

This chapter describes certain patterns of pain that aid in making a diagnosis. Some of the common acute conditions, such as shock and hemorrhage, peritonitis, and bowel obstruction, are reviewed, and following this the causes of acute abdominal pain are grouped according to their major characteristics.

SHOCK AND HEMORRHAGE

The circulation is maintained by the cardiac pump, the blood volume, the resistance of arterioles in the peripheral circulation, and the reservoir capacity of the veins. In shock the effective circulation is decreased and tissue perfusion becomes inadequate. The four major types of shock are hypovolemic, septic, neurogenic, and cardiogenic.

Hypovolemic shock may result from loss of whole blood by hemorrhage, or loss of electrolytes and plasma by bowel obstruction, peritonitis, severe vomiting and diarrhea, or thermal burns. Loss of blood volume causes a decrease in venous pressure and a decrease in volume of venous blood returned to the heart. In response the heart increases its rate, and arterioles in nonvital areas, such as skin, muscle, and splanchnic circulation, constrict. The result is preservation of coronary and cerebral circulation at the expense of all others. This shift in circulation is the first mechanism to compensate for discrepancy between the volume of circulating blood and the capacity of the blood vessels.

If further compensation is needed to counteract shock, several reactions occur to maintain blood volume. As renal circulation decreases, renal filtration and urine output decrease. Decreased renal artery pressure stimulates renin production. Renin stimulates aldosterone secretion by the adrenal cortex, which causes water and salt retention. Renin also stimulates angiotension II release causing vasoconstriction and an increase in blood pressure. Perhaps the most important compensation of all occurs in the capillary circulation. The decreased pressure of the arteriolar inflow discourages loss of fluid from capillaries by reduction of hydrostatic pressure. The resorption of fluid at the venous end of the capillary remains normal because the serum proteins are unaltered. The result is an increase in absorption of fluid from the interstitial fluids to the blood stream. In turn water moves from the cells to the interstitial fluids and a degree of intracellular dehydration occurs. Movement of interstitial fluid into the blood stream begins as soon as hypovolemia occurs, whereas intracellular fluid movement occurs more slowly.

Mild shock could be defined as a loss of less than 20% of blood volume, equivalent to a hemorrhage of less than one liter. As a rule the reaction to this loss is a change in distribution of blood flow. There is a decrease in circulation to nonvital parts, such as the skin and skeletal muscle. Decreased skin circulation causes a feeling of coldness, and the skin is gray looking, pale, and cool to the touch. Decreased circulation to skeletal muscle produces weakness and prostration. The body temperature is lower. The patient is aware of danger, clear minded, but anxious and frightened. The pulse rate may be mildly increased.

Moderate shock may be defined as a loss in blood volume between 20 and 40%. The reaction to this loss is a decrease in perfusion of viscera, such as intestine, kidneys, and liver. The pulse is more rapid and less forceful. Systolic blood pressure is lower and urine volume decreases. Muscular weakness is profound; the patient is apathetic and may be drowsy. He or she feels thirsty and may develop nausea and vomiting. Body temperature drops. On examination there is evidence of dehydration. Drop in systolic blood pressure is the main clinical sign that shock is uncompensated.

Severe shock is associated with a loss of effective blood volume greater than 40% of normal. When this occurs, there is a decrease in circulation to the lungs, heart, and brain. The pulse is even more rapid and weak and the blood pressure is low. The skin circulation is sluggish and the skin appears mottled, ashen, and cyanotic. The patient may be restless and agitated, may have the panting respirations of air hunger, and may become sleepy or semiconscious. There is severe thirst. Cardiac irregularity and coma are serious developments.

Septic shock is associated with septicemia, most often caused by infection by gram-negative organisms. Capillary permeability increases, which allows loss of fluid into extravascular tissues. Blood vessels are relaxed, their resistance is lowered, and the blood pressure falls. The infection may produce a toxic effect on the heart. There is a discrepancy between the volume of the vascular space and the fluid available to fill it. When the patient is hypovolemic and septic shock ensues, the clinical picture resembles hypovolemic shock. The patient has cold, pale skin, low cardiac output, and low central venous pressure. When the patient develops septic shock while normovolemic, cardiac output is increased, the skin is warm and dry, and the central venous pressure may be normal or high. In both cases there is oliguria, hyperventilation, and mental confusion. Normovolemic septic shock might occur in a patient after rupture of an abscess. Hypovolemic septic shock might complicate bowel obstruction, strangulation, or perforation. Patients with either variety of septic shock may develop progressive pulmonary insufficiency, hypoxia, and respiratory alkalosis (1).

Neurogenic shock occurs with decreased peripheral resistance resulting from inhibition of sympathetic tone in blood vessels. Inhibition of vasoconstrictors can occur for a variety of reasons, such as severe pain, fear, a horrid sight, removal of a cast or sutures, spinal cord injury, quadriplegia, or spinal anesthesia. The effective blood volume is decreased as blood pools in veins. Lowering the head improves venous return to the heart and this may be sufficient to treat shock. Neurogenic shock is caused by vasodilatation.

Cardiogenic shock is caused by decreasing cardiac output because of weakening of the cardiac pump. Central venous pressure increases as blood is backed up in the venous side of the circulation. Peripheral resistance in arterioles increases to maintain circulation to the myocardium and brain. The heart pump may weaken because of coronary occlusion, arrhythmia, other myocardial disease, or severe valvular disease.

When hypovolemic shock occurs because of loss of electrolyte solution or plasma, the proportion of cells to fluid in the blood stream rises. Blood cell count, hemoglobin concentration, and hematocrit are increased. Electrolyte solutions given intravenously cause hemodilution and reduce these values toward normal. When bleeding occurs the loss of serum is proportional to the loss of blood cells. At first blood cell counts, hemoglobin, and hematocrit are normal, but when redistribution of fluid occurs and electrolyte solutions are given intravenously, these values drop as the circulating blood becomes dilute.

Blood in the peritoneal cavity is an irritant. However, the shock associated with intraperitoneal hemorrhage is caused by the blood loss and hypovolemia rather than the peritoneal irritation.

A small amount of blood slowly entering the peritoneal cavity is rapidly diluted by a transudate and remains unclotted, but a larger more rapid hemorrhage into the peritoneum clots. Clotted blood around a bleeding organ and unclotted blood in remote parts of the peritoneum allow the clinician to detect fixed dullness over the bleeding organ and remote shifting dullness as characteristic physical signs. During a laparotomy for intraperitoneal hemorrhage, the bleeding site is likely to be where the clots are found. If clotting is normal, the recovery of nonclotting bloody fluid from abdominal tap is evidence that the bloody fluid is from the peritoneal cavity and that intraperitoneal bleeding has taken place.

The major shock mechanisms are:

Venous return failure: Hypovolemia, venous vasodilatation

Inadequate cardiac filling: Pleural, mediastinal, and pericardial tamponade

Failure of pump action: Myocardial disease, arrhythmias, valvular failure

Cardiac outflow obstruction: Pulmonary embolus, mediastinal tamponade, pleural tamponade, dissecting aortic aneurysm

Decreased peripheral resistance: Arteriolar vasodilatation, arteriovenous shunting, severe sepsis, severe pain

ACUTE PERITONITIS

The peritoneum is a large, collapsed bursal sac capable of prompt response to irritation. The first reaction is transudation of fluid. In this reaction the irritant might be diluted and spread about so that there is a greater surface available for absorption. Leukocytes and antibodies rapidly enter the peritoneal cavity in response to infection. Irritants may be localized by the various peritoneal pouches, inflammatory adherence of one structure to another, adhesions, and the omentum. The unattached portion of the normal omentum can drift freely in the peritoneal cavity. Whenever it touches an area of inflammation, it becomes attached by fibrin, and because of its circulation, the omentum forms another route for leukocytes and proteins to reach the inflamed area.

As a rule peritonitis is secondary to an inflamed abdominal organ. Perforation may occur, but bacteria can migrate through inflamed bowel wall. Chemical irritants induce an effusion at first, but eventually bowel organisms produce an infection. Peritonitis may be caused also by penetrating wounds and by hematogenous infections. In primary peritonitis, which is rare, the bacteria may reach the empty peritoneal sac by the bloodstream or by migration through the female genital tract.

Since acute peritonitis is most often caused by spread of infection from an inflamed abdominal organ, the early history and clinical findings in acute peritonitis are those of the original inflammation. When the infection spreads to the peritoneal surface, usually requiring an hour or two, there is an increase in the intensity and extent of the local pain and tenderness. Peritonitis may be described in four stages.

The first stage is the stage of intramural inflammation where the infection is confined to the wall or substance of the abdominal organ. The main symptom is a poorly localized visceral pain that begins insidiously and is not severe. The pain is not associated with neurogenic shock. On examination the patient may not look ill, although the temperature and pulse may be elevated, and shows no sign of bleeding, shock, or dehydration. The only abdominal finding is tenderness over the inflamed organ. There may be direct tenderness and sometimes direct rebound tenderness but usually no remote tenderness. If this visceral pain is severe it may be associated with referred pain and occasionally reflex spasm of nearby body wall muscles.

The second stage of peritonitis occurs as infection spreads to the parietal peritoneum. Adjacent organs and omentum become adherent and tend to localize the infection. A clearer, sharper, better localized pain begins at the site of the inflammation. This deep somatic pain appears whenever the inflammation spreads to the parietal peritoneum or root of the mesentery. On examination the patient looks ill and both the temperature and pulse rise. The abdomen moves very little with respiration. There may be hyperesthesia and guarding over the site of inflammation. Muscle guarding may prevent deep palpation. There is direct tenderness, percussion tenderness, remote tenderness, and as a rule both direct and remote rebound tenderness. Reflex contraction of regional muscles is found. Referred pain may be felt in another area supplied by the same spinal nerve. Muscles that are held in reflex contraction may become tender and painful, another reason for regional pain and tenderness. There may be fever, malaise, weakness, pallor, prostration, and fear. The patient may perspire and have nausea and vomiting. There is leukocytosis, a higher proportion of immature granulocytes, and a more rapid erythrocyte sedimentation rate. Movement produces pain so that the patient prefers to remain supine and still and to breath shallowly.

The reaction to the local peritonitis may bring about resolution of the infection, or an abscess may form. The pus is held locally by the adherence of organs and omentum and may produce a palpable mass. As a rule pain lessens as the inflammation becomes localized. The appetite is poor and the bowels are constipated unless the abscess lies in the pelvis in which case the rectum is irritated, there is regional hyperemia, and diarrhea occurs. On examination the patient does not look ill or dehydrated, but there is fever and tachycardia, the rigidity has disappeared, and a tender and immobile mass with indistinct edges may be felt. Leukocytosis and increased sedimentation rate persist.

The fourth is the stage of diffuse peritonitis. Inflammation may have penetrated the wall of the abdominal organ so quickly that there has been no time for localizing reactions to occur. Diffuse peritonitis occurs when an abscess ruptures into the peritoneal cavity. Instead of a well-localized pain, there is diffuse severe parietal pain over the whole abdomen. The patient looks ill and shows signs of dehydration. The eyeballs are soft and sunken, the cheeks hollow, the tongue dry and furred, and the skin inelastic. Anxiety, pain, and dehydration are the reasons for the sunken-cheeked, staring appearance often seen in patients with advanced peritonitis. The distended abdomen is held immobile. The entire abdominal wall may be hyperalgesic. Deep palpation is prevented by the tenseness of the distension and muscle rigidity. There is resonance on percussion and the bowel sounds disappear. Dehydration occurs because of loss of fluid into the peritoneal cavity, perspiration, and vomiting.

PERFORATION

Perforation of an abdominal viscus can occur because of penetrating wounds, crush injury, disease of hollow organs, perforation by a swallowed foreign body, or complication of an obstruction. Following a penetrating injury it is necessary to investigate for perforation of a hollow viscus and for intraperitoneal bleeding. Similarly a severe crush injury to the abdomen requires investigation for possible rupture of an intra-abdominal organ or hemorrhage. The physician should try to evaluate the pain and tenderness produced by the injury to the abdominal wall and then concentrate on signs of possible intra-abdominal complication.

The commonest disease that causes perforation is duodenal ulcer. A mixture of acid gastric juice, pancreatic juice, and bile produces severe chemical irritation of the peritoneum. When a duodenal ulcer perforates, the transudation of fluids into the peritoneal cavity in response to the chemical irritation is early and massive. Hypovolemic shock of severe degree occurs and may cause death.

Uninfected dilute bile is a mild irritant and unactivated pancreatic juice is nonirritating. Achlorhydric gastric juice associated with perforated gastric carcinoma is a mild irritant to the peritoneum. Urine is irritating according to the degree of infection. Small bowel contents are irritating according to the potency of enzymes and bacterial pathogenicity. Colonic contents are always infected and are highly irritating; perforation of the colon always causes acute inflammation. Leakage of an abdominal abscess or perforation of obstructed intestine produces a flood of highly infected fluid into the peritoneal cavity and acute diffuse peritonitis.

Pain is the main symptom of a perforation. The main characteristic of the pain of a perforation is that it either starts or ceases abruptly (5). Sudden flooding of the peritoneal cavity produces sudden, severe, diffuse abdominal pain, so severe that it causes neurogenic shock. The patient becomes immobile, is frightened to move, perspires freely, feels nauseated, and may vomit. As the irritant becomes diluted or neutralized the pain may improve. On the other hand, if the perforation follows an obstruction, the pain prior to the perforation increases in severity up to the time of perforation. Suddenly the distended organ is decompressed as perforation occurs. The pain abruptly lessens, and soon acute peritonitis develops.

On examination patients hold themselves immobile and are distressed and pale. There are no signs of dehydration or hemorrhage unless these complicate the injury or disease causing perforation. Fever begins as peritonitis develops. The abdominal wall does not move with respiration because of widespread muscular rigidity. There is no distension unless the perforation has been present for a period of time. Bowel sounds cannot be heard. Plain X-rays may show gas in the peritoneal cavity.

The clinician must remember almost one-fourth of the abdominal cavity lies within the pelvis, and the innervation of the pelvis has no representation in the muscles of the anterior and lateral abdominal walls. The irritant must spread upwards out of the pelvis to produce extensive rigidity of the abdominal wall muscles. Almost one-third of the abdominal cavity lies under the costal margins, which can be examined only with difficulty. Irritation in this part of the abdominal cavity may be associated with abdominal wall rigidity or both abdominal wall and intercostal muscle rigidity.

PARALYTIC ILEUS

Paralytic ileus is a functional paralysis of the muscle of the gastrointestinal tract. It is not a primary condition but is always secondary to injury, abdominal disease, or disturbance somewhere else in the body. It may be localized to a short segment of the intestinal tract near an inflamed organ, but more often it is widespread. Effective peristaltic action is suppressed and the bowel becomes paralyzed; neither feces nor gas is passed by rectum. The stomach passively distends with swallowed air and accumulated gastric juice. Gas in the paralyzed bowel causes distension at all levels. Bowel sounds that are normally heard every 20 seconds become infrequent or disappear completely. Regurgitant vomiting occurs. If the patient is elderly or the pharyngeal reflexes are paralyzed, there is danger of pulmonary aspiration. Pain is not necessarily a feature. The main discomfort is that of abdominal distension. There may be hiccups and shallow breathing. There is intractable constipation.

The most common cause of paralytic ileus is acute peritonitis. Other causes include anesthesia; laparotomy; abdominal injury; severe abdominal pain, such as renal colic, twisted ovarian cyst, biliary colic; disease of extra-abdominal organs, such as pneumonia, myocardial infarction, renal infections, uremia, fractures of ribs, spine, or pelvis; biochemical disturbances such as potassium depletion or chronic morphine poisoning; and mesenteric vascular occlusion. Acute gastric dilation and postoperative urinary retention are related conditions. The causes of paralytic ileus are categorized as:

Infection: Intra-, extra-, and retroperitoneal sepsis; gastrointestinal perforations; pneumonia

Hemorrhage: Intra-, extra-, and retroperitoneal bleeding

Surgery: Operations, anesthetic agents, vagotomy

Drugs: Anticholinergics, ganglion blocking agents, narcotics
Metabolism: Hypokalemia, alkalosis, uremia
Reflex: Trauma, fractures of spine and pelvis, back injuries, severe pain and shock
Hypoxia: Mesenteric vascular insufficiency; infarcts of spleen, kidney, omentum, or heart

On examination the patient lies quietly in little distress yet does not appear well. There are no distinctive appearances. The abdomen is distended and tympanitic on percussion. Tenderness and rigidity may be present if the paralytic ileus is caused by peritonitis. No intestinal peristaltic sounds are heard. The heart sounds are heard with cavernlike clarity. Other signs depend upon the cause. Similarly laboratory results depend upon the duration of the primary condition, the degree of infection, and the dehydration. Plain X-rays usually demonstrate gas in all portions of the gastrointestinal tract. Relatively more gas than fluid is seen as compared with mechanical bowel obstruction. One or several adjacent loops of bowel may be distended with gas, and lie beside an inflamed organ. These are called sentinel loops and their position suggests the probable cause of the paralytic ileus.

The resumption of peristaltic activity signals recovery from paralytic ileus. Active bowel sounds, passage of gas by rectum, and relief of abdominal distension are signs of effective peristalsis.

Paralytic ileus after trauma to the abdomen suggests that there has been intraperitoneal hemorrhage, a perforated viscus, or other visceral injury. Secondary disappearance of peristaltic activity after early recovery of peristalsis following an operation must be considered serious. As a general rule this indicates the onset of peritonitis which may be caused by anastomotic leak. Sudde cessation or sudden onset of abdominal pain suggests a perforation and t' suspicion is confirmed by the onset of paralytic ileus and peritonitis.

The sudden onset of severe, steady visceral pain accompanied by sl and paralytic ileus suggests a strangulation. Torsion of an ovarian cyst common cause. The intestine may undergo strangulation without a prec mechanical obstruction. This happens with interference of intestinal flow by mesenteric vascular occlusion or insufficiency. The stages of mes vascular occlusion are:

Neurogenic shock: Visceral pain, mesenteric vasospasm
Hypovolemic shock: Somatic pain, mesenteric vasodilatation, mucos tion, edema, and hemorrhage
Septic shock: Acute peritonitis

Sudden onset of diarrhea, which is usually bloody, occurs soon after nset ction of regional pain. Occasionally, especially in the left colon, ischemic occurs instead of the more common hemorrhagic infarction of bowel. In this case profuse diarrhea without blood occurs as a result of sudden occlusion of the inferior mesenteric artery.

MECHANICAL INTESTINAL OBSTRUCTION

In mechanical obstruction of the bowel the lumen is occluded as opposed to paralytic ileus where there is no occlusion. The onward passage of intestinal content is blocked, and the bowel above the obstruction increases its peristaltic contractions in force and frequency to overcome the obstruction. The bowel above the obstruction becomes distended with accumulated fluid and gas; the distal bowel soon empties itself.

Intestinal obstruction alters the fluid and electrolyte exchanges in the bowel; fluid is lost by vomiting; and the bowel distal to an obstruction is no longer available for absorption. Water and electrolytes accumulate above the obstruction. The increase in hydrostatic pressure within the bowel proximal to the obstruction decreases absorption, and this leads to further accumulation of fluid above the obstruction. As intraluminal pressure increases, the circulation to the bowel wall becomes impaired.

Complete obstruction of the bowel causes crampy abdominal pain, vomiting, abdominal distension, and obstipation. The crampy pain is caused by increased peristalsis above the obstruction. This is associated with hyperactive bowel sounds. Cramps arising from the midgut are periumbilical and from the hindgut, hypogastric, in location. Abdominal distension occurs because of the dilated bowel proximal to the obstruction. One or occasionally two bowel movements may occur after the onset of obstruction as the bowel distal to the obstruction empties, but after that neither feces nor gas is passed by rectum. There is forceful vomiting in contrast to the effortless vomiting of paralytic ileus. The causes of intestinal obstruction are summarized as follows:

Luminal: Fecal impaction, food bolus, worms, polypoid tumor, foreign body, gallstone, intussusception

Mural: Atresia, stricture, paralytic ileus, tumor, diverticulitis, regional ileitis, carcinomatosis

External: Adhesions, tumor, hernia, abscess, volvulus

In incomplete bowel obstruction some of the accumulated fluid passes
ough the narrowing. Although there is crampy abdominal pain and often
e abdominal distension, diarrhea occurs. Incomplete obstruction is fre-
tly confused with acute gastroenteritis, but the order of onset of the
res is different. The usual sequence in acute gastroenteritis is nausea and
ing, then crampy abdominal pain, no distension, and finally diarrhea. In
lete bowel obstruction the usual sequence is crampy abdominal pain,
on, vomiting, and infrequent diarrhea.

All four characteristics of complete bowel obstruction, crampy pain, abdominal distension, vomiting, and obstipation, are not present in every case. If one considers the prominence and the time of onset of each, one can determine the level of obstruction with some accuracy. The earlier the onset of vomiting the higher the obstruction. The extreme in this case is the regurgitation of each swallow with esophageal obstruction. Crampy pain does not occur with obstruction at or proximal to the pylorus. The early onset of crampy pain suggests small bowel rather than colonic obstruction. Similarly early distension of the abdomen is greater the more distal the level of obstruction. The more distal the obstruction, the shorter the length of bowel that can empty after the onset of the obstruction. Immediate obstipation occurs with sudden onset rectal obstructions. As a rule the longer the interval between cramps, the lower the obstruction (Table 5).

The general effects of an obstruction are caused by loss of water and electrolytes. Dehydration and hypovolemia cause thirst, weakness, and prostration. Dehydration is the main disturbance in esophageal obstruction. In pyloric obstruction the effects of vomiting are dehydration, alkalosis, and hypokalemia. Below this level vomiting results in loss of gastric juice and small bowel secretions. Small bowel secretions have electrolyte concentrations similar to their concentrations in plasma. In all cases hypovolemia leads to uremia.

The vomitus in esophageal obstruction is swallowed material and saliva. The vomitus in pyloric obstruction is sour gastric juice mixed with swallowed food and fluid but no bile. In upper small bowel obstruction the vomitus also contains bitter green bile. Malodorous, orange-colored, stagnant small bowel contents indicate a well-established low small bowel obstruction. Feculent, not fecal, vomitus is caused by bacterial decomposition in the small bowel (Table 6).

On examination the patient is distressed by episodes of crampy pain and

Table 5 Causes of Intestinal Obstruction According to Age and Level of Obstruction

Age group	Cause
Newborn	
high	Atresia, volvulus, meconium ileus
low	Imperforate anus, Hirschsprung's disease
Infants	
high	Congenital adhesions, strangulated hernia
low	Intussusception, Hirschsprung's disease
Adults	
high	Adhesions, carcinomatosis, hernia
low	Carcinoma, volvulus
Elderly	
high	Carcinomatosis, hernia, gallstone ileus
low	Carcinoma, diverticulitis, fecal impaction

Table 6 Characteristics of Intestinal Obstruction According to the Level of Obstruction

Area	Vomiting	Cramps	Distension	Obstipation
Esophagus	Every swallow or two, food and saliva	None	None	Late
Pylorus	Large volume, old food, no bile, once daily	None	Epigastrium, succussion splash	Late
Jejunum	Earlier than ileal	Initial symptom, severe	Mild or none	After colon is empty
Ileum	Later than jejunal	Initial symptom, severe	Moderate, central	After colon is empty
Proximal colon	Later	Second symptom	Initial symptom, severe	After distal colon is empty
Rectum	Late	After distension appears	Second symptom, massive	First symptom, tenesmus

vomiting but is fairly comfortable in the intervals. Soon thirst and electrolyte disturbance cause weakness and prostration. Severe distension of the abdomen occurs in lower bowel obstruction, but distension is less obvious in high small bowel obstruction. The epigastrium may be full and there may be a succussion splash demonstrable in pyloric obstruction just before vomiting.

If the abdominal wall is thin, peristaltic waves may be seen with bowel obstruction. As a rule peristaltic waves seen in patients with colonic obstruction are caused by small bowel peristalsis. Hyperactive bowel sounds accompany visible peristalsis and crampy pain. All hernial orifices must be palpated for a mass or tenderness. A search is made for a tumor mass. Auscultation reveals the gurgling sounds of gas and fluid churned by hyperactive peristalsis. The percussion note is resonant over gas-filled bowel.

The pulse, blood pressure, and temperature are normal at first. Dryness of the tongue and lips, soft sunken eyeballs, and loss of tissue turgor are found. Dryness causes hemoconcentration. The hemoglobin, hematocrit, and blood cell count are above normal. Plain X-rays of the abdomen with the patient erect or in the lateral decubitus position reveal gas–fluid levels in the small bowel where normally no gas is seen. Plain X-ray of the abdomen with the patient supine shows the extent of gas-filled bowel. If the obstruction is complete, little or no gas is seen below the obstruction. If gas is seen by X-ray at all levels in a case of clinically diagnosed mechanical obstruction, it means the obstruction is incomplete; it does not mean that the clinical diagnosis is incorrect and the patient has paralytic ileus. The distended jejunum may be seen in the upper central abdomen with mucosal folds crossing the bowel from one side to the other. The distended ileum tends to lie centrally in the lower abdomen with a flatter, smoother outline. The colon lies peripherally and shows the bulging of the haustrations, but the folds between haustrations do not pass completely across the bowel. The largest gas-filled segment of bowel, or the longest air–fluid level, in the right lower quadrant is the cecum. When the ileocecal valve is competent, the cecum bears the brunt of colonic distension and is the part that perforates as a rule. In colonic obstruction rectal, sigmoidoscopic, and barium enema examinations are used to demonstrate the obstruction. Barium is not given by mouth to demonstrate small bowel obstruction unless the obstruction is clearly incomplete.

The high risk types of intestinal obstruction are:

Paralytic ileus: Intraperitoneal hemorrhage, ruptured viscus, intestinal strangulation, undrained abscess

Mechanical ileus: Unresolved mechanical obstruction, strangulated hernia, closed loop obstruction

INTESTINAL OBSTRUCTION WITH STRANGULATION

Primary intestinal strangulation is associated with paralytic ileus. In this category are mesenteric vascular occlusion, retroperitoneal hemorrhage or tumor, and low flow in splanchnic circulation. Secondary intestinal strangulation is a complication of mechanical intestinal obstruction in the form of unresolved mechanical obstruction, closed-loop obstruction, or colonic obstruction. It occurs more rapidly than uncomplicated obstruction as a rule and is more serious.

In closed-loop obstructions there is double occlusion of the bowel. The mesenteric veins may be compressed. The bowel wall swells, and fluid accumulates in the segment. The proximal obstruction must be incomplete if air is found in the segment; more often the loop is filled with fluid alone. The pressure within the loop and on the mesenteric veins causes impaired circulation in the bowel walls. As swelling increases, hemorrhagic infarction occurs. Bacteria and blood seep through the wall of the strangulated bowel, and frank perforation is the fatal next step.

Double- or closed-loop obstruction may occur when a loop of bowel is caught in a hernia or in a volvulus. When the ileocecal valve is competent, colonic obstructions are closed loop. The closer the colonic obstruction is to the cecum, the more rapid is the distension of the cecum and the greater the danger of early perforation. Unrelieved mechanical bowel obstruction runs the danger of strangulation when the distension becomes severe.

The clinical presentation includes the features of mechanical intestinal obstruction with tenderness over the obstructed segment, local peritoneal irritation, and shock. At first the shock is neurogenic because of severe pain, then hypovolemic because of fluid losses and redistribution, and finally septic when perforation occurs. There is steady pain as well as cramps. There is pain, tenderness, rebound tenderness, and guarding over the strangulation. A tender mass is an extremely important discovery. Thirst and vomiting are early and severe. There is general weakness, prostration, and fear of impending disaster.

The patient appears to be in distress exhibiting pallor, cold perspiration, rapid breathing, weak and rapid pulse, and low blood pressure. The temperature is low at first, but fever appears as infection becomes established. The hemoglobin and hematocrit may drop because of blood loss, but the leukocyte count rises because of infection. X-ray reveals nothing characteristic of strangulation, although swollen bowel wall suggests edema or hemorrhage, either of which may be caused by strangulation.

It is difficult to differentiate nonstrangulating from strangulating obstruction. However, strangulation is suspected where the onset of the obstruction is rapid; the pain, tenderness, and rigidity are severe; fever and leukocytosis are found; and the patient appears to be quite ill and in shock.

The clinical presenation and findings may show that more than one type of obstruction is present. In fact as mechanical obstruction becomes established the nearby proximal bowel fatigues and dilates, and peristalsis becomes ineffective. Similarly hyperactive peristalsis may be found proximal to the region of bowel immobilized by paralytic ileus. Both paralytic ileus and mechanical obstruction can be complicated by strangulation. Nevertheless, if the patient is studied to determine the order of appearance of the various features, a correct diagnosis on clinical grounds can be made in most cases.

Diagnosis by Pattern Analysis

The first chapter described the clinician's ranking of diagnostic possibilities according to frequency, seriousness, treatability, and novelty (4). The frequency of the causes of serious pain in patients seeking help varies from one region to another and according to the place where help is sought, ranging from the primary care physician's office to a large general hospital with facilities to provide ultimate care in all specialties. The frequency of the causes of abdominal pain in patients seeking help in the Casualty Department at the General Infirmary in Leeds, England is shown in Table 7 (3). The frequency of diseases associated with abdominal pain leading to emergency admission of adults to St. Michael's Hospital, Toronto is shown in Table 8 (6).

SUDDEN ONSET ABDOMINAL PAIN

All of the conditions associated with a sudden or abrupt onset of abdominal pain are the result of mechanical events. These events include perforation and rupture of normal and abnormal abdominal structures; torsion of pedunculated structures; hemorrhage into the peritoneal cavity, retroperitoneum, or abdominal

Table 7 Emergency Examinations for Acute Abdominal Pain in Casualty Department of The General Infirmary, Leeds, England[a]

Cause	%
No significant disease	50
Acute appendicitis	20
Acute cholecystitis	9
Perforated duodenal ulcer	5
Small bowel obstruction	4
Acute pancreatitis	2
Acute diverticulitis	2
Other	8

[a]From (3).

wall; and vascular occlusion caused by thrombosis or embolism (Figure 15). A more detailed list includes:

Perforation: Duodenal ulcer, sigmoid diverticulitis, esophagus, gastric ulcer, obstructed bowel, typhoid or tuberculous ulcer of small bowel, amoebic ulcer of colon, toxic megacolon

Rupture: Abscess, hematoma, cyst

Torsion: Testis, ovary, volvulus of small or large bowel, omentum, appendices epiploicae

Hemorrhage: Leaking, dissecting, or other aneurysm, ectopic pregnancy, spleen, rectus sheath, rupture of pregnant uterus, blunt trauma, rupture of hematoma

Infarction: Infarct of intestine, spleen, kidney, lung, heart

Table 8 Adult General Surgical Admissions for Acute Abdominal Pain, St. Michael's Hospital, Toronto[a]

Cause	%
Acute appendicitis	24
Acute cholecystitis	21
Acute diverticulitis	17
Bowel obstructions	16
Acute pancreatitis	8
Perforated ulcer	5
Other	9

[a]From (6).

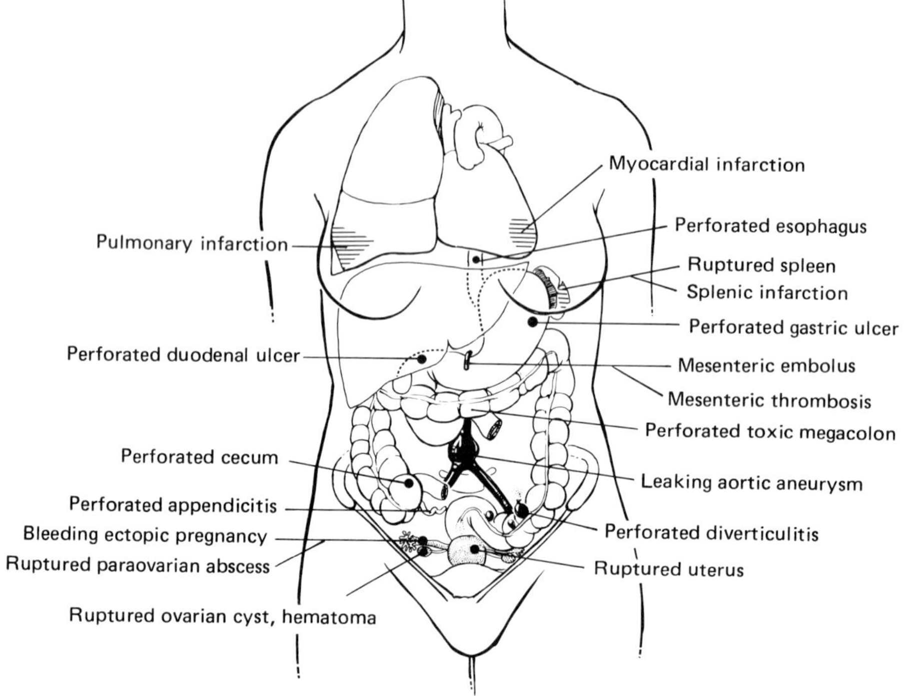

Figure 15 Some causes of sudden onset abdominal pain. Among other causes not shown are rectus sheath hematoma, torsion or volvulus of intestine, and torsion of the testis.

The severity and seriousness of perforation or rupture depends upon the nature and amount of material released through the disruption. Highly irritating fluids cause severe pain, rapid loss of fluid into the peritoneum, and early onset of hypovolemic shock. The signs of peritonitis are easily demonstrated soon after the leakage. Spillage of highly infected fluid from obstructed or diseased bowel or from an abscess is complicated by septic shock. Leakage of blood from a laceration or rupture of the spleen, ectopic pregnancy, or rupture of the pregnant uterus causes hypovolemic shock.

Sudden onset or sudden cessation of pain is typical of perforation. Similarly a sudden onset of acute peritonitis is suspected of being caused by a perforation or leakage. Intraperitoneal rupture of a structure containing gas is diagnosed by the X-ray demonstration of free air in the peritoneal cavity where there is no other cause, such as recent laparotomy, culdoscopy, or laparoscopy. Absence of free air does not rule out a perforation.

Torsion of an abdominal structure is a cause for abrupt onset abdominal pain. Twisting can occur only when the structure has one or two narrow attachments. Volvulus of small bowel, cecum, or sigmoid colon is a serious complication because it is a closed-loop obstruction. Torsion blocks venous return so that congestion and swelling are found. Eventually hemorrhagic infarction occurs. Volvulus of the small bowel is more prone to strangulation than volvulus of the colon. In volvulus of the colon gas readily accumulates in the loop and is easily recognized on plain, supine X-rays of the abdomen. Volvulus of the small intestine infrequently contains gas.

A vascular occlusion causes infarction of part or all of the tissues supplied exclusively by the blocked blood vessel. The severity varies from transient ischemia to frank gangrene depending on the collateral circulation, the duration of the ischemia, and the rate of occlusion. If the vascular occlusion is sudden, the bowel goes into violent spasm. The regional vessels also undergo spasm. After a short time the anoxic muscle relaxes, the unblocked vessels dilate, the part becomes congested, the mucosa secretes profusely, and watery or bloody diarrhea appears. If the occlusion is more gradual the pain from the initial spasm is less severe. The treatment and its success vary with the severity and duration of the ischemia prior to diagnosis.

As a rule the more sudden the onset and the more severe the degree of abdominal pain, the more urgent the need for surgical care. Delay is tragic. Almost invariably, abrupt onset of abdominal pain means a surgical emergency.

The causes of abdominal pain of rapid onset include not only the causes of abrupt onset of abdominal pain, such as perforation, rupture, torsion, hemorrhage, and vascular occlusion, but also blockage of tubular structures and inflammations that develop rapidly. It is clear that any of the causes of abrupt onset may unfold more gradually because of adherent structures, less severe disease, less potent infection, incomplete torsion, slower hemorrhage, less extensive thrombosis, small embolus, and better collateral circulation (Figure 16).

Blockage of the ureter or small intestine may produce rapid onset abdominal pain. Impaction of a stone in the upper ureter causes the steady pain of renal colic in the kidney region. Small bowel trapped in a hernia or small bowel obstruction resulting from twisting or distortion by adhesions causes abdominal pain to develop quickly. Similarly intussusception, gallstone ileus, and other less common causes of small bowel obstruction usually develop rapidly. Blockage of the cystic duct by a gallstone causes biliary colic and later, acute cholecystitis if the blockage persists and infection supervenes. If infection does not occur a mucocele results.

Inflammation of abdominal organs may develop rapidly. Some cases of appendicitis, salpingitis, and diverticulitis appear so quickly that the correct diagnosis is not considered initially. Although pancreatitis probably begins as a chemical inflammation, it often appears so quickly that it needs to be included in the causes of rapid onset abdominal pain. Pneumothorax, pneumonia, and pleurisy often begin more precipitously than one would ordinarily expect.

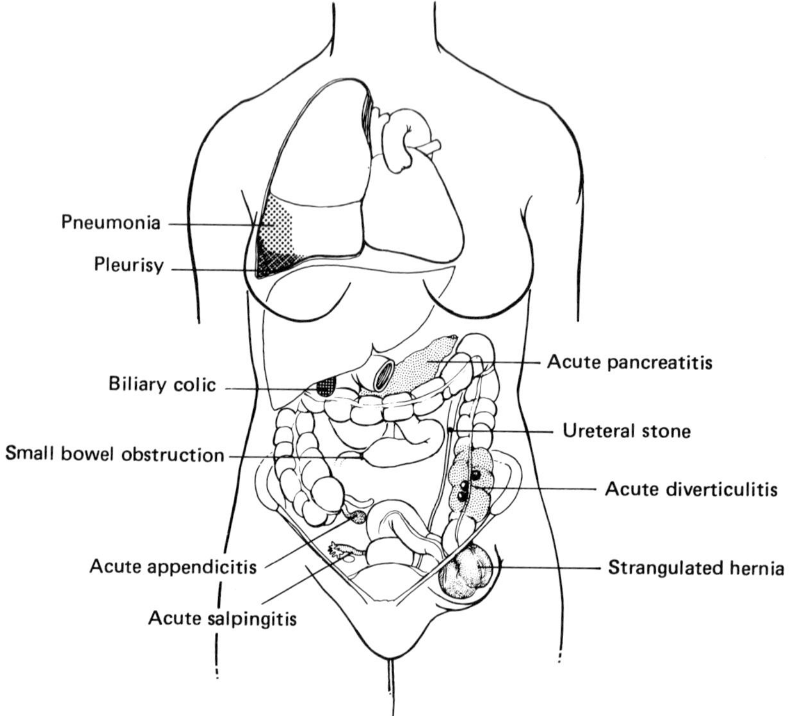

Figure 16 Some causes of rapid onset abdominal pain. Many of the conditions in Figure 15 could be included in this category if the onset were less than abrupt. Similarly some of these conditions could begin suddenly.

STEADY ABDOMINAL PAIN WITH PERITONEAL IRRITATION

The causes of steady abdominal pain with peritoneal irritation are:

Peritonitis: Penetrating wounds, appendicitis, diverticulitis, salpingitis, bowel perforation, abscess rupture, postoperative infection, anastomosis leakage
Hemorrhage: Spleen, ectopic pregnancy, ruptured aneurysm, trauma
Perforation: Peptic ulcer, malignant ulcer, trauma, pancreatic pseudocyst

Steady abdominal pain with peritoneal irritation comprises all of the causes of acute peritonitis. The clinical picture results from peritoneal irritation, paralytic ileus, and the systemic effects of the inflammation. The severity of the disease is caused by the intensity of the irritation, the virulence of the infection, the amount of fluid lost into the peritoneal cavity, the resistance of the patient to infection, and the duration of the disease. Treatment is always more effective the earlier it is begun. The principles of treatment include resuscitation, removal of the irritant, stopping the leakage, drainage, and treatment of the disease. Often resuscitation can be no more than started before other measures are needed. Removal of the irritant may include operative and occasionally post-operative peritoneal lavage. The leakage may be stopped by patching a perforated peptic ulcer, removing the appendix or gallbladder, resection of bowel, diversion of the fecal stream, repair of lacerations, removal of tubal pregnancy or ruptured spleen, or aortoiliac grafting.

Serious peritonitis often develops from localized disease. Abdominal pain, tenderness, and muscle guarding must be watched carefully lest the irritant spreads without recognition. Especially dangerous is the relief of abdominal pain of an inflamed organ as it ruptures. Unless the patient is examined repeatedly, this change will be missed. Examples of this are acute appendicitis, acute cholecystitis, and intra-abdominal abscess.

STEADY ABDOMINAL PAIN WITHOUT PERITONEAL IRRITATION

Steady pain in the abdomen without peritoneal irritation, or before peritoneal irritation is evident, is caused by infection, ischemia, extraperitoneal hemorrhage, retroperitoneal inflammation, or infiltration. Abdominal pain may be caused by distension of a hollow organ because of obstruction to the outflow or by disease of the wall. Distension caused by outflow obstruction occurs in biliary colic, renal colic, and prostatic obstruction with urinary bladder distension. Distension from abnormality within the wall of a hollow organ includes enlarging aortic aneurysm and paralytic ileus. Gastric dilatation and postoperative urinary retention are common in the early postoperative period. Steady abdominal pain without initial peritoneal irritation is also caused by torsion of the omentum, an ovarian cyst, or the testis. Ischemia is another cause for steady abdominal pain without peritoneal irritation in the early stages as is hemorrhage into the walls of the aorta with dissecting aneurysm, into the retroperitoneal tissues with leaking aortic aneurysm, or into the rectus sheath with spontaneous rupture of an inferior epigastric artery.

As long as the inflammation is confined to the organ, acute pancreatitis, pyelonephritis, hepatitis, salpingitis, pelvic inflammatory disease, and lymphadenitis cause steady abdominal pain but no peritoneal irritation.

Infiltration of a malignant tumor produces steady, usually unrelenting pain without peritoneal irritation. The earliest symptom of pancreatic carcinoma is steady, aching pain, and its main characteristic is its steady, unrelenting nature, provided that allowance is made for distraction of the patient's attention and the effects of analgesics. Continuous pain at night may be the best clue. As a rule an enlarging aortic aneurysm is more episodic. Either of these two conditions may cause abdominal or back pain.

CRAMPY PAIN WITHOUT ABDOMINAL DISTENSION

Crampy abdominal pain without distension is almost synonymous with crampy abdominal pain resulting from causes not associated with intestinal obstruction. Crampy pain or colic in the abdomen arises only from the intestine and the uterus; one must distinguish intermittent steady pain such as the pain of an enlarging aortic aneurysm, repeated splenic or renal infarcts, or repeated torsions of omentum, an ovarian cyst, or other female adenexal structures. All of the nonmetabolic or nontoxic causes of intestinal cramps without distension are caused by inflammation of the walls of the small or large intestine. These include bacterial and viral gastroenteritis, chronic ulcerative colitis, regional ileitis, and other forms of enteritis and colitis. These diseases are usually characterized also by diarrhea. When the inflammation rests mainly in the midgut, the cramps are felt in the umbilical region, rarely on the right side. When the disease affects primarily the descending and sigmoid portions of the colon, the cramps may be felt in the hypogastrium or occasionally on the left side of the abdomen. If one carefully questions patients having sigmoid colon cramps, one usually finds that the pain is felt in the hypogastrium. However, once the patient realizes the pain is associated with tenderness in the left lower quadrant, the patient then often says that the crampy pain is felt in the left lower quadrant rather than in the middle of the hypogastrium.

Ureteral or renal colic is almost invariably unilateral and on the same side as the cause. These pains are steady, similar to biliary colic, and are caused by obstruction and distension. Pain resulting from renal pelvic or upper ureteric obstruction is felt in the costomuscular angle in the back; obstruction of the lower ureter can cause back pain and groin pain.

Uterine crampy pain is felt during menses and delivery. Threatened abortion is characterized by little pain and little vaginal bleeding, but inevitable abortion is expected when there is moderate or severe uterine cramps, moderate vaginal bleeding, and dilatation of the cervix.

Other causes of crampy abdominal pain without distension include metabolic disturbances such as diabetic acidosis and porphyria, and heavy-metal poisoning with lead, arsenic, or mercury.

Crampy abdominal pain is a visceral pain. Cramps from the intestine may occur in the early stages of appendicitis, bowel obstruction, intestinal strangulation, or other serious disease. For this reason it is important to keep patients having visceral pain under observation. If not examined repeatedly, such patients may develop diffuse peritonitis before again seeking help. Similarly steady abdominal pain may be the visceral pain of the early stages of acute cholecystitis, pancreatitis, or appendicitis. Again all patients having visceral pain must be examined repeatedly.

CRAMPY ABDOMINAL PAIN WITH DISTENSION

Probably the most common cause of attacks of intestinal cramps with distension is the irritable colon syndrome—constipation type with gas bloat. Malabsorption is an uncommon cause for abdominal cramps and distension. Uterine cramps with distension is usually easily distinguished from intestinal cramps with distension on clinical examination alone. In all other cases abdominal crampy pain with abdominal distension indicates bowel obstruction, which may be either complete or incomplete and may result from a wide variety of causes:

Small bowel obstruction: Adhesions, carcinomatosis, hernia, volvulus, intussusception, Meckel's diverticulum, gallstone ileus

Colonic obstruction: Carcinoma, diverticulitis, volvulus, fecal impaction, ischemic stricture

Other: Spastic colon with gas bloat, malabsorption

It is helpful to list the causes of acute abdominal pain arising from diseases other than disease of the gastrointestinal tract according to the characteristics of the abdominal pain:

Intestinal cramps: Poisoning, porphyria

Steady pain: Leukemia, sickle-cell anemia

Pain and shock: Leaking or dissecting aortic aneurysm, myocardial infarction

Neuralgic pain: Spinal nerve compression, herpes zoster, spinal cord tumor

Bizarre pain: Diabetic ketoacidosis, periarteritis nodosa, lupus erythematosus

Abdominal wall muscle spasms: Heat stroke, adrenal crisis, hypocalcemia, arachnidism, neurological disease with spasticity

ABDOMINAL PAIN ACCORDING TO SITE

It may seem too elementary to consider pattern recognition of abdominal pain according to site as most physicians know the location of abdominal organs. However, pain may occur in areas other than the usual position of abdominal organs (Figure 17).

The central midepigastrium is the site of visceral pain arising from structures derived from the embryonic foregut and from intrathoracic structures supplied by branches of the lowest seven thoracic nerves. Common lesions include biliary colic, acute pancreatitis, peptic ulcer, acute gastritis, myocardial ischemia, and diffuse esophageal spasm. Cramps in the midepigastrium alone are very rare and probably arise only from obstruction in the short segment

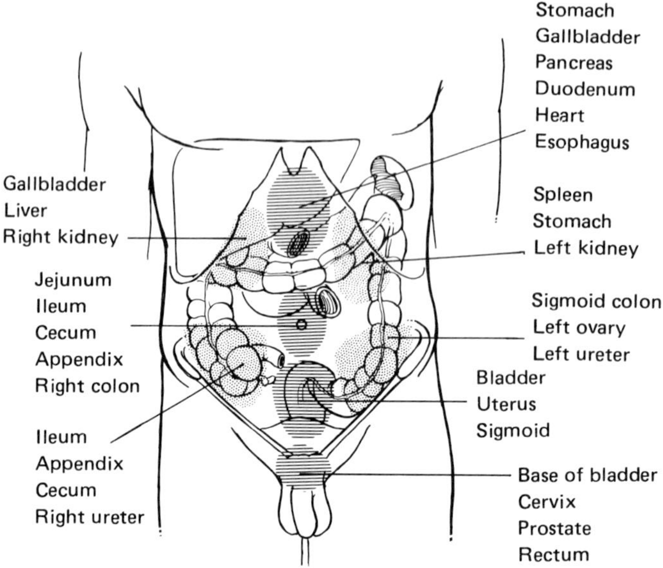

Figure 17 Abdominal pain according to site. Visceral pain occurs mostly in the midline. Patients who have visceral pain must be examined repeatedly because parietal pain, local tenderness, and other signs may develop that will reveal the underlying condition.

of the duodenum at or proximal to the duodenal papilla. Epigastric hernia is an abdominal wall cause for pain in this region.

The central umbilical region is the site of visceral pain from structures derived from the embryonic midgut. In general, cramps indicate an intestinal irritation or obstruction, and steady pain suggests a strangulation or closed-loop obstruction. Visceral pain from the appendix is usually crampy; steady umbilical pain from the appendix suggests closed-loop obstruction and the risk of early perforation. Severe, steady umbilical pain and shock suggests superior mesenteric artery embolus or thrombosis or aortic aneurysm. The umbilicus itself should be carefully examined for disease that may cause pain.

Central hypogastric or suprapubic pain may arise from the proximal hindgut or from pelvic structures. The most common reason for suprapubic pain is distension of the urinary bladder. Since the sigmoid colon is free of the posterior peritoneum, visceral pain from the sigmoid colon is usually felt in the midline of the hypogastrium. Visceral pain from the body of the uterus may be felt in the suprapubic region also. Although the innervation of the fallopian tubes and ovaries is unilateral, these structures are close to the midline and pain arising from these structures may be felt in the middle or near the middle of the hypogastrium. Acute salpingitis and pelvic inflammatory disease are usually bilateral and pain is experienced in the midline of the suprapubic or pelvic regions in these cases.

Pain arising in the anterior abdominal wall may be caused by abdominal wall hernia, rectus sheath hematoma, muscle cramps associated with heat stroke, or muscle spasms during the first day after laparotomy. Entrapment neuropathy is a possible cause of pain arising in the abdominal wall. Relief with local anesthetic injection confirms the source of the pain.

Pain arising in the posterior abdominal wall may be caused by collapsed vertebra; secondary tumor of the spine; extruded lumbar intervertebral disc; expanding, leaking, or dissecting aortic aneurysm; or a large number of less common causes. Pain in the sacral region may be caused by local disease, such as secondary tumor in the sacrum, by disease of organs derived from the primitive cloaca. Thus acute cervicitis, prostatitis, proctitis, and neoplasms in these regions may produce pelvic and posterior midsacral pain. Pilonidal sinus infection is a local obvious cause for posterior sacral pain.

Right upper quadrant abdominal pain results from parietal peritoneal irritation and is commonly caused by diseases of the gallbladder or liver. Swelling of the liver causes right upper quadrant abdominal pain rather than epigastric pain because of the liver's attachment to the parietal peritoneum. The right upper abdomen may be the site of pain arising from the right kidney. Tenderness of the kidney may be demonstrated by pressing in the right costomuscular angle posteriorly and in the right upper abdominal quadrant anteriorly. Other causes of right-sided upper abdominal pain are liver abscess, rapid enlargement of the liver, and subhepatic or subphrenic abscess.

Left upper quadrant abdominal pain is less common. Acute splenitis, acute splenic enlargement, splenic infarction, and several gastric lesions cause left upper abdominal pain. Gastric tumor, acute gastritis, and gastric ulcer are examples. Pain from the left kidney is an occasional cause of pain in the left upper quadrant of the abdomen.

Right lower quadrant abdominal pain is common, and the most common organic cause is acute appendicitis. Right lower quadrant abdominal pain is felt when inflammation in the appendix extends outward to irritate the nearby parietal peritoneum. Other painful lesions in this region include acute ileitis, regional ileitis, obstruction of the ascending colon causing cecal distension, and disease of the right ovary.

Left lower quadrant abdominal pain is common in the elderly because the frequency of diverticulosis and its complications increases with age. Acute diverticulitis is the most common cause of left lower abdominal pain and tenderness in the elderly. Obstructing and infiltrating tumors of the sigmoid colon occasionally cause pain. Because the descending colon is applied to the posterior abdominal wall, visceral pain from the descending colon may be felt on the left side of the abdomen rather than in the middle of the hypogastrium. Sudden onset, steady left lower quadrant abdominal pain with shock and diarrhea with or without bleeding suggests inferior mesenteric artery occlusion.

The transverse colon resembles the sigmoid colon in that it does not lie against the posterior parietal peritoneum. The transverse colon is derived from the midgut, and visceral pain is felt in the umbilical region.

TROPICAL DISEASE AND ABDOMINAL PAIN

Tropical diseases may be grouped according to the abdominal quadrants they affect. Tropical diseases causing right upper quadrant abdominal pain include amoebic abscess, acute hepatitis, suppurative myositis, oriental cholangiohepatitis, hookworm infestation resulting in duodenitis and pain, ascaris infestation of the bile ducts, and enlarging or infected hydatid cyst of the liver. In the left upper quadrant of the abdomen splenic enlargement from malaria, splenic Leishmaniasis (Kala-azar), and splenic infarction related to sickle-cell disease may cause pain. In the right lower quadrant of the abdomen amoebic colitis, tuberculous or typhoid ulceration of the ileum, and intussusception are causes of abdominal pain. In the left lower quadrant amoebic colitis may cause abdominal pain. Volvulus of the sigmoid colon is a cause of pain in the abdomen, most of which is attributable to intestinal obstruction of the volvulus (Figure 18).

Diffuse abdominal pain may occur in the tropics because of worm infestation, heat prostration causing muscle cramps, giardiasis, and salt deficiency secondary to unreplaced loss of salt from excessive perspiration. Severe

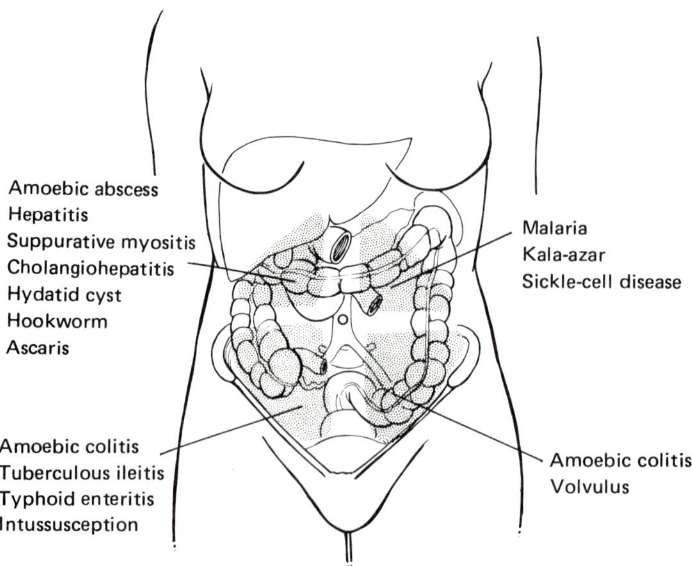

Figure 18 Tropical diseases according to abdominal quadrant.

muscle pain may be caused by leptospirosis, dengue, trichinosis, malaria, or Coxsackie virus infection.

POSTOPERATIVE ABDOMINAL PAIN

After operations on the abdomen pain is usually confined to the region of the incision, and after the first day it is mostly related to movement. Respirations are shallow since deep inspiration causes pain. The pulse is rarely over 100 per minute, and fever is not expected in the postoperative period. In the first 36–48 hours after operation peristalsis is disorganized and ineffective, and bowel sounds are rarely heard. Sudden severe pain of brief duration caused by sudden contraction of abdominal wall muscles is not unusual in the first 24 hours. The danger signs in the early postoperative patient include persisting pain, tachycardia, rapid respirations, abdominal distension, fever, leukocytosis, general toxicity, and prolonged paralytic ileus or secondary disappearance of bowel sounds after postoperative resumption.

Allowance must be made in evaluating the postoperative condition of the very elderly and the very young. Similarly patients on immunosuppressive medication and adrenocorticosteroid hormones may show deceptively mild responses to serious complications especially to infection. Healing may be greatly delayed.

Complications of the incision include bleeding, dehiscence, and infection. Hematoma may be extensive especially if the tissues are soft and a pressure dressing is not used. The lax tissues in the elderly and the loose tissues of the axilla, scrotum, and neck allow more bleeding than firmer tissues. Patients receiving anticoagulants may have extensive bleeding. A sudden strain, such as an unexpected cough or sneeze, may break a recently sutured wound. One of the first signs of abdominal wound dehiscence is the appearance in a previously dry wound of a quantity of pink watery fluid from the peritoneal cavity. If the muscle and fascia are not resutured, one must expect an incisional hernia. Wound infections do not appear for three or four days unless the operative field included a highly infected area. Wounds that become painful and ischemic after an initial period of relative comfort and good circulation may be developing necrotizing fasciitis, a surgical emergency.

Accidental injury to internal organs at the time of surgical operation is a rare cause of postoperative pain. It is bad enough to cause injury to organs; it is much worse not to recognize the injury and repair it immediately. Friable organs, such as the spleen and the colon, may be injured by retractors or in dissections made difficult by adhesions. Any operation near the ureters must include their methodical display and protection. Difficult dissection of the ureters should be anticipated; their identification is greatly aided by preoperative insertion of ureteral catheters by cystoscopy. The gallbladder, appendix, and, in adults, the spleen should be removed if major injury occurs.

Anastomotic leaks are relatively unimportant if the area is well drained, there are no signs of peritonitis, and the patient remains well. Healing of the fistula occurs unless there is a distal obstruction, foreign body, fecal impaction, discontinuity of bowel, reinfection, neoplasm, or idiopathic inflammatory disease of the bowel remaining at the site of the fistula.

Leakage of an undrained anastomosis is far more serious and difficult to recognize. The secondary disappearance of bowel sounds after their postoperative return is a very important observation. Tachycardia, abdominal distension, fever, abdominal tenderness, and increasing volume of drainage from nasogastric suction are important signs. Unless serial films are taken, X-ray demonstration of free air in the peritoneum caused by anastomotic leakage is difficult to distinguish from free air remaining in the peritoneal cavity after laparotomy. It is seldom safe to administer contrast media for X-ray demonstration of leakage except for rupture of the esophagus. All enemas are contraindicated when perforation of the colon is suspected.

An early complication may be postoperative hemorrhage. Tachycardia, hypotension, pallor, and oliguria despite transfusion of blood in sufficient volume to replace operative losses make the diagnosis obvious. Any bleeding or clotting mechanism deficiency must be corrected. Postoperative hemorrhage severe enough to cause hypovolemic shock despite adequate transfusion usually requires immediate reoperation. Prolonged postoperative pain may be the initial clue to this complication.

Postoperative bowel obstruction is difficult to recognize. It should be suspected with abdominal distension following the reappearance of bowel sounds. Such an obstruction may be caused by a swollen anastomosis, a loop of bowel caught in a suture used to close the abdominal incision, a volvulus, or an internal hernia. Bowel may be obstructed if a loop passes through a suture line, such as the closed pelvic peritoneum or the abdominal incision. Often repeated examinations and serial plain X-rays of the abdomen are needed to recognize these obscure complications. Unexplained hypovolemia, renal failure, hypotension, and jaundice should suggest postoperative acute pancreatitis. It may follow any abdominal operation but is most common after operations on the pancreas and bilary tract or for duodenal ulcer disease. The mortality of postoperative acute pancreatitis is high (2). Elevated serum amylase concentration is helpful in recognizing this complication. If detection of this complication is late, the urine amylase concentration remains elevated longer than the serum amylase concentration and may be a more useful sign.

Postoperative complications can be difficult to recognize. Repeated clinical examination, awareness of the more common complications and a deliberate search for such complications are part of the safe management of patients following any surgical operation. The earlier these complications can be recognized the earlier and therefore the more successful they can be treated.

Pattern recognition can be a most helpful method in diagnosis of the causes

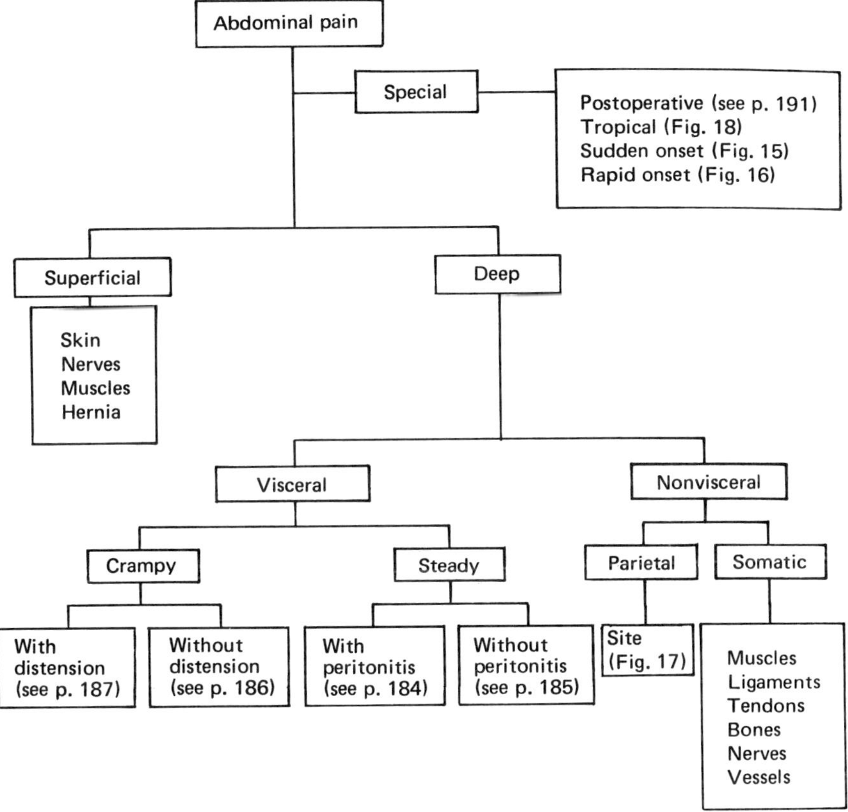

Figure 19 An approach to the problem of diagnosis of abdominal pain.

of abdominal pain. One approach to the problem of diagnosis by pattern recognition is shown in Figure 19. This method in one form or another is used by most clinicians.

REFERENCES

1. Artz CP, Cohn I, Davis JH: Brief Textbook of Surgery. Philadelphia: Saunders, 1976.
2. Botsford TW, Wilson RE: The Acute Abdomen, 2d ed. Philadelphia: Saunders, 1969.
3. DeDombal FT: Computer-aided diagnosis and decision-making in the acute abdomen. J R Coll Physicians Lond 9:211–218, 1975.
4. Elstein AS, Kagan N, Shulman LS, Jason H, Loupe MJ: Methods and theory in the study of medical inquiry. J Med Educ 47:85–92, 1972.

5. Perkins G: The Foundations of Surgery. Edinburgh: Livingstone, 1954.
6. St. Michael's Hospital, Toronto, Medical Records, 1977.

FURTHER READING

Dunphy JE, Way LW: Current Surgical Diagnosis and Treatment. Los Altos, Calif: Lange, 1973.

Gelin L, Nyhus LM, Condon RE: Abdominal Pain. Philadelphia: Lippincott, 1969.

Jones PF: Emergency Abdominal Surgery in Infancy, Childhood and Adult Life. Oxford: Blackwell, 1974.

Lowenfels AB: Companion Guide to Surgical Diagnosis. Baltimore: Williams & Wilkins, 1975.

Passmore R, Robson JS: A Companion to Medical Studies. Oxford: Blackwell, 1974.

Shepherd JA: A Concise Surgery of the Acute Abdomen. Edinburgh: Churchill, Livingstone, 1975.

Shepherd JA: Surgery of the Acute Abdomen, 2d ed. Edinburgh: Livingstone, 1968.

Chapter 9

Systemic Diseases with Abdominal Pain and Other Problems

A number of patients have abdominal pain resulting from systemic conditions. A history of recurring episodes, a prolonged illness recently complicated by abdominal pain, or unexpected systemic symptoms may be the first clue that systemic rather than abdominal disease is the cause of the abdominal pain. Some patients have abdominal pain as the most prominent feature, but in others the features of the systemic disease predominate.

Systemic signs, such as fever, sweating, weakness, dehydration, leukocytosis, and increased sedimentation rate, are found with any infection. However, beware of unusually high fever, chills or rigors, profuse diarrhea, pain and stiffness in a number of joints, and skin eruptions. Pay attention to chest, cardiac, urinary, or gynecological symptoms and signs, such as dyspnea, pleurisy, productive cough, urethral or vaginal discharge, and bloody or dark urine. Watch for lymphadenopathy, splenomegaly, joint swellings, skin rashes, hepatomegaly, and abnormal neurological signs. When the abdominal signs are minimal but the distress appears to be great, beware of a medical cause especially if the patient is young (6, 11). Systemic or medical diseases are discussed below.

ENDOCRINE DISORDERS

Diabetes Mellitus

When patients with diabetes mellitus develop metabolic ketoacidosis, a few complain of abdominal pain sufficiently severe to create a diagnostic problem. The cause of the pain is not known. Most patients with this problem are young, insulin-dependent, and in ketoacidosis with serum bicarbonate levels under 10 milliequivalents per liter (2). Correction of the ketoacidosis coincides with relief of the pain. Abdominal pain caused by diabetic ketoacidosis is less likely in older patients; so other causes should be expected in patients over 40 years of age. Young uncontrolled diabetics may complain of nausea and vomiting and steady or crampy pain. They are dehydrated and may be drowsy. There is little abdominal tenderness and no rigidity of abdominal wall muscles. The initial step with all diabetics must be to bring the diabetes under control as quickly as possible. The urine must be tested for the presence of glucose and ketones in every patient undergoing investigation for abdominal pain. Serum amylase level should be determined because diabetic ketoacidosis with abdominal pain may be associated with acute pancreatitis.

Acute abdominal complications may precipitate ketoacidosis in a diabetic patient. When diabetes is diagnosed in an elderly patient with vague, constant, epigastric pain, the possibility of carcinoma of the pancreas should be considered. Carcinoma of the pancreas is common in established diabetics. Intestinal angina is very rarely encountered, but diabetes mellitus is common in these patients. Similarly type I or V hyperlipoproteinemia may be present in patients with intestinal angina, probably caused by postcibal hyperviscosity of the serum.

Adrenal Insufficiency

Adrenal crises may be caused by sudden drug withdrawal after long-term steroid administration, trauma, anticoagulant therapy, bilateral adrenal necrosis and hemorrhage usually associated with fulminant infections (Waterhouse-Friderichsen syndrome), and a number of other causes. There may be central abdominal pain and unexpected vascular collapse, nausea, vomiting, and diarrhea. Serum sodium, chloride, and glucose concentrations are low and blood urea nitrogen and potassium concentrations are elevated. The plasma 11-hydroxycorticosteroids are greatly reduced and do not rise with adrenocorticotrophic hormone stimulation. Eosiniphilia may be found. These laboratory tests should be done before treatment is started in mild cases. However, in severe cases treatment with corticosteroids must be begun on clinical suspicion alone because these rare conditions can be fatal within hours.

Many patients with either primary or secondary adrenal insufficiency produce enough corticosteroids for basal requirements but are unable to meet the increased requirements of stress. The stress of an abdominal complication, a fluid overload after operation, an infection, or myocardial infarction may precipitate adrenal insufficiency and create a difficult differential diagnosis.

Hyperparathyroidism

Hyperparathyroidism may be associated with acute pancreatitis, troublesome constipation, and duodenal ulceration because of stimulation of hydrochloric acid secretion. Hypercalcemia causes skeletal muscle weakness, anorexia, nausea, and vomiting. There may be a history of renal stones, bone pain, or pathological fracture. Personality changes, most frequently chronic depression, are common. These patients are sometimes discovered during investigation of poor response to psychotherapy.

Hypocalcemia

Hypocalcemia, especially if associated with hypomagnesemia, and low serum sodium are often found with skeletal muscle cramps. Hypocalcemia may cause severe muscle spasm, tetany, and laryngeal stridor.

Hyperthyroidism

Hyperthyroidism may be associated with intermittent diarrhea because of hyperperistalsis, abdominal cramps, nausea, and vomiting. Skeletal muscle weakness is common.

Hypothyroidism

Hypothyroidism may occur with severe constipation and, in the elderly, fecal impaction with abdominal pain. Ascites and pleural and pericardial effusions are not uncommon.

METABOLIC DISORDERS

Acute Intermittent Porphyria

Acute intermittent porphyria is inherited as an autosomal dominant trait. It affects females slightly more commonly and is more common in Sweden. The abdominal pain is crampy, abdominal tenderness is less than expected for the intensity of the pain, and there is vomiting and constipation. The urine turns deep red on exposure to light. During an attack the patient may be confused or at times psychotic and occasionally convulsive. The motor impairment ranges from minor weakness to quadriplegia and even bulbar palsy and death (10). The diagnosis is made by a positive test for urinary porphobilinogens, which is specific for acute intermittent porphyria. Many of these patients have multiple laparotomy scars.

Hyperlipoproteinemia

Hyperlipoproteinemia (type I) is an extremely rare familial abnormality of infants or children, inherited as an autosomal recessive and is often associated with hepatomegaly and splenomegaly. Acute pancreatitis may be the first indication of the disease. Episodes of pancreatitis and other features of the disease resolve on a low-fat diet. Pancreatitis with severe chylomicronemia can also occur occasionally in an older person secondary to alcoholism, diabetic ketoacidosis, myxedema, and dysglobulinemia.

Mediterranean Fever

Mediterranean fever is a rare familial disorder inherited as an autosomal recessive in patients from the Mediterranean region. These patients have a history of recurrent bouts of fever, polyserositis, and acute abdominal pain. The abdominal pain is associated with peritonitis. Often there is pleural effusion, joint swelling, erythema, splenomegaly, and later, perhaps, amyloidosis. There is no diagnostic test.

Angioneurotic Edema

Angioneurotic edema is a rare familial autosomal dominant condition characterized by localized edema. Especially dangerous is laryngeal edema. The abdominal pain is associated with submucosal edema, peritoneal effusion, and no sign of inflammation. Nausea, vomiting, and abdominal cramps are caused by submucosal swelling. A deficiency of C1-esterase, a component of complement, is diagnostic.

Hemochromatosis

Hemochromatosis is an uncommon disease of men, sometimes complicated by acute abdominal pain and tenderness. There is an increase in iron absorption with a steady accumulation of iron in the body over a number of years. The iron deposition in the liver, heart, and endocrine organs leads to cirrhosis, cardiac enlargement, cardiac failure, and gonadal atrophy. Unexpected right-sided abdominal pain may result from a hepatoma; one patient in seven may be expected to have this complication. Biopsy of the liver and the effects of phlebotomy establish the diagnosis.

Uremia

Uremia may be associated with much nausea and vomiting, diffuse abdominal pain, tenderness, and distension. One should suspect uremia whenever vomiting, diarrhea, or paralytic ileus appear without an apparent cause.

INFECTIOUS DISEASES

Acute Gastroenteritis

Acute gastroenteritis is caused most commonly by the ingestion of pathogenic organisms that have been excreted in the feces. It is characterized by chills, high fever, dehydration, and profuse diarrhea. Stool specimens examined by smear and culture may identify *Shigella spp.*, *Salmonella spp.*, or enteropathogenic *E. coli*, but the majority are caused by viruses.

Acute Hepatitis

Acute hepatitis is characterized by severe anorexia and malaise, nausea, vomiting, right upper quadrant dull aching pain, tender hepatomegaly, diarrhea, and jaundice.

Infectious Mononucleosis

Infectious mononucleosis may be associated with diffuse steady or right lower quadrant abdominal pain and tenderness as a result of swollen mesenteric lymph nodes. This condition should be suspected in young adults having unexplained fever and lymph node enlargement. The spleen and occasionally the liver may be enlarged and tender. The predominance of mononuclear cells in a blood smear and a positive sheep-cell agglutination test confirm the diagnosis.

Herpes Zoster

Herpes zoster is a reactivation of a chickenpox viral infection of a posterior root ganglion that may cause spinal nerve pain before the vesicular chickenpox rash appears in the affected dermatome.

Nonspecific Mesenteric Lymphadenitis

Nonspecific mesenteric lymphadenitis often begins with symptoms and signs of an upper respiratory infection in a child or young adult. Right lower quadrant abdominal tenderness results from tender, swollen mesenteric lymph nodes.

Often the point of tenderness is not as discrete and is more medial than in early appendicitis, but the differentiation can be impossible. As a rule there is no preceding periumbilical visceral pain from the midgut in nonspecific mesenteric lymphadenitis as there is in typical acute appendicitis.

HYPERSENSITIVITY DISEASES

Rheumatic Fever

Rheumatic fever may be associated with bouts of diffuse abdominal pain. At times fibrositis of the abdominal wall or serositis may be recognized. Fever, polyarthritis, pericarditis, chorea, subcutaneous nodules, nosebleeds, and skin rash form the clinical picture. Abdominal pain may be diffuse or more localized to the region of the small bowel mesentery where the lymph nodes appear to be responsible for the tenderness.

Henoch-Schonlein Purpura

Henoch-Schonlein purpura may be associated with pain and tenderness in the abdomen. Purpuras or hematomas may develop in the bowel wall because of capillary fragility, and gastrointestinal bleeding may occur. The bowel changes may initiate an intussusception. Joint pains, fever, papular and petechial rashes, and normal platelet concentration are features. Abdominal cramps occur in about 50% of the children and young adults affected.

Lupus Erythematosus

Lupus erythematosus may be linked with abdominal distension and peritoneal effusion. One should suspect systemic lupus erythematosus when fever, rash, anemia, polyarthritis, pleuritis, pericarditis, and murmurs occur. Inflammation of serosal surfaces leads to polyserositis including peritonitis. Diarrhea, intestinal ulceration, hemorrhage, or perforation may occur. A positive antinuclear factor test in high titer and lupus erythematosus cells in the peripheral blood support the diagnosis.

Periarteritis Nodosa

Periarteritis nodosa is associated with bizarre pain and tenderness in any organ. Acute pancreatitis is not unusual in young adult males with this disease. Intestinal infarction and peritonitis may occur. Fever, hypertension, hematuria, albuminuria, edema, peripheral neuritis, weakness, and weight loss are the main features. Diagnosis may be established by biopsy of any tissue that contains an inflamed artery.

POISONS AND TOXINS

Heavy-Metal Poisoning

Heavy-metal poisoning is associated with severe gastroenterocolitis. Lead poisoning causes crampy abdominal pain simulating obstruction. Vomiting occurs and loud bowel sounds are heard. Diarrhea may not be prominent; in fact there may be constipation. Neuritis, wrist or foot drop, reflex changes, lead line, basophilic erythrocyte stippling, and anemia are found. Lead poisoning is proven by finding a high concentration of lead in the urine. Severe gastro-enteritis follows the ingestion of arsenious oxide. Mercurial poisoning results in severe colitis.

Arachnidism

Archnidism is caused by the bite of a black widow spider, *Latrodectus mactans,* and is characterized by diffuse severe pain and rigid muscles that are tender. Abdominal pain is caused by sustained contraction of muscles of the abdominal wall. Pain, swelling, and redness are found at the site of the bite. Dizziness, weakness, pain in the extremities, and shock may occur.

Oxalic Acid

Oxalic acid ingestion causes abdominal cramps and diarrhea; rhubarb tops or green apples in quantity are sources.

HEMATOLOGICAL DISEASES

Sickle-cell Disease

Sickle-cell disease causes sudden sharp stabbing abdominal pain. Red blood cells clump and plug small vessels, causing microinfarcts. Right upper quadrant pain may be caused by liver congestion. In children and adolescents left upper quadrant abdominal pain is produced by splenic infarcts. Most of the symptoms are generated by microinfarcts in various parts of the body. The patient is usually black and has chronic anemia and joint pain. The wet paraffin-rimmed coverslip smear of blood allows identification of sickled erythrocytes. Patients of black ancestry with abdominal pain must be tested for sickle-cell disease.

Polycythemia and Leukemia

Polycythemia and leukemia cause left upper quadrant abdominal pain because of splenic infarcts. These infarcts usually heal and form adhesions between the spleen and the diaphragm. Thrombocytopenia is a frequent accompaniment.

Hemophilia

The retroperitoneal hemorrhage of hemophilia causes abdominal pain. Retroperitoneal bleeding in the right lower quadrant of the abdomen may confuse the clinical picture with acute appendicitis.

Lymphoma

Lymphoma may cause pain by bowel obstruction or infiltration into any abdominal organ or tissue. Mesenteric lymph nodes enlarge, lymphatics become blocked, and chylous ascites may be found.

RECURRENT ABDOMINAL PAIN IN CHILDREN AND ADOLESCENTS

The majority of children having recurrent abdominal pain do not have an organic abnormality. Approximately 1 child in 10 will be found to have a physical cause for recurrent abdominal pain. Most of these physical abnormalities become apparent on clinical examination and can be supported by a few appropriate investigations. It is mandatory to take a complete history and perform a thorough examination (5). Watch for gastrointestinal and genitourinary abnormalities (1). In young girls especially a urinary tract infection may be associated with bizarre symptoms and may be easily missed unless a midstream urine specimen is carefully collected and studied (4). Constipation must be eliminated as a possible cause for recurrent abdominal pain. Pinworms cause perianal itching and occasionally abdominal pain. They may be found on the skin at the anus or the ova may be found in the stools. Stool examination for occult blood might be the initial sign of intestinal polyps or Meckel's diverticulum. Also watch for upper respiratory tract infection and tonsillitis without throat complaints. Periodic illnesses, such as migraine and epilepsy, may be associated with recurrent abdominal pain, but the relationship is not clear.

In the majority of cases clinical examination reveals little evidence for organic disease but positive evidence for stress-induced distress. The family history of a child with recurrent abdominal pain often discloses a notable familial prevalence of peptic ulcer, recurrent headaches, nervous breakdown, or recurrent abdominal pain of childhood persisting into adult life. The incidence of family discord is high. Some children copy the abdominal pain of a close friend or relative who is ill or of an older sister who has severe menstrual cramps. Recurrent abdominal pain may be the childhood equivalent of recurrent headaches in adults. One must determine whether the child feels emotionally, intellectually, or physically inadequate at school, with friends, or at home with the family.

Once the problem is identified it must be presented to the parents in such a way that it will be fully accepted. The parents must be convinced of the explanation and be willing to participate in their child's management. Only then will one of Dr. Apley's "little bellyachers" be helped (1).

For a very few cases exploratory laparotomy might be considered the practical solution because of persisting or recurrent complaints and repeated periods of absence from school. Before exploratory operation is undertaken all of the investigations described above must be completed, as well as an intravenous pyelogram to rule out a genitourinary abnormality and a barium enema to rule out colonic polyps or malrotation as possible causes. Often this operation is limited to a right lower quadrant oblique incision since this quadrant is the most frequent site of recurrent abdominal pain. Appendectomy and exploration of the ovaries and distal ileum are necessary parts of this operation.

PARAPLEGIA AND QUADRIPLEGIA

Spinal cord injury usually results in a variable period of spinal shock characterized by loss of sensation and voluntary movement and by depression of reflex activity at and below the level of injury. The bony injuries are recognized by X-ray examination and the neural damage is diagnosed by clinical investigation. Spinal shock is associated with loss of sympathetic vasomotor tone. Peripheral resistance is reduced as arterioles relax; blood pools in dilated veins. The result is arterial hypotension and relative hypovolemia caused by expansion of the vascular capacity. The manifestations are generally reversible if the patient is tilted head downward.

As the period of spinal shock passes, reflex activity returns at levels lower than the injury wherever the spinal reflex arc is intact. The long tracts that are physically divided or destroyed do not recover, and there is permanent loss of superficial, deep, and visceral sensation; loss of voluntary motor activity; and hyperreflexia with release of suprasegmental inhibition. Extensor plantar reflexes may be found at this stage.

Reflex motor activity tends to reappear first in flexor muscles. Stimulation can cause widespread muscle contractions that might include incontinence of the bladder and bowel, a mass reflex. Extensor reflexes return later; so there is a tendency for the patient to hold most joints in flexion. Active physiotherapy is needed to prevent flexion deformities.

With return of flexor motor activity there is return of smooth muscle reflexes. Apart from a short period of paralytic ileus following the injury to the spinal cord, intestinal reflexes continue without interruption; intestinal reflexes are unique in that they are independent of the spinal cord. Some form of neurogenic bladder takes place. Tachycardia occurs with cervical lesions, and bradycardia occurs with high thoracic lesions. Sweating, hypertension, and changes in pulse rate may be problems at first but subside with time.

Many spinal cord injuries and diseases result in partial destruction of the long tracts. These patients may retain some superficial, somatic, or visceral sensation and some voluntary motor activity. Abnormalities of reflex activity are not difficult to detect. A careful study of the anatomy of segmental innervation and an appreciation of the completeness of the cord lesion leads to an understanding of the reactions in most cases. A study of paraplegics and quadriplegics with lesions at various levels and with different degrees of spinal cord destruction has helped greatly in understanding visceral sensation.

In spinal injury patients with absence of parietal pain sensation disease of abdominal organs can progress to serious complications with few symptoms and signs. Remember that the undersurface of the diaphragm is innervated by the phrenic nerve. Thus shoulder-top pain is the highest segmental innervation for pain from the parietal peritoneum; otherwise there is no parietal pain from the abdomen. Pain from disease in the foregut can be appreciated despite a complete cord lesion above the C3 segment because some visceral pain is transmitted by the vagus nerves (3).

In patients with lesions above T5 painful abdominal conditions provoke a complaint of a vague and variable amount of visceral pain. There is increased activity of autonomic reflexes: sweating of the face, neck, and arms above the neural lesion; hypertension; tachycardia; fever; anorexia; and often nausea, vomiting, and headache. The abdominal wall may be rigid in the absence of peritoneal inflammation because of general spasticity of skeletal muscles. On the other hand the abdominal muscles may relax despite peritonitis (9). Some patients have bladder spasms and diarrhea; yet others have paralytic ileus and abdominal distension.

As the abdominal disease progresses to involve the parietal peritoneum, most patients with intact sensation are able to localize the pain to the appropriate segment. Patients with incomplete lesions can localize the site of disease earlier and more accurately. Patients with cord lesions below T7 can localize their abdominal disease earlier than patients having lesions at higher levels because they have better abdominal sensation. Those with cord lesions below T7 are more likely to have tenderness, rebound tenderness, and abdominal wall muscle guarding. Tenderness and guarding are important in these patients. Reduced or absent bowel sounds always mean paralytic ileus, and this may be the most useful sign of abdominal disease or injury in these patients. If pain is sharp and radicular in distribution, consider a neurological lesion as the cause of the pain (7). Root irritation at the level of injury is the most frequent cause of pain in a paraplegic; pain from an upper urinary tract infection is the next most frequent (8).

Abdominal disease is difficult to assess in patients with cord lesions, and unfortunately treatment is often delayed. Pay special attention to the patient with a spinal cord lesion who feels that something is wrong; has nausea or vomiting, headache, loss of appetite; becomes unexpectedly restless; and develops fever, tachycardia, and hypertension. Increased activity of intact spinal reflexes below the level of the lesion may occur. Absence of bowel sounds and abdominal distension are important signs. Hypotension following a period of distress and elevated blood pressure may indicate a serious complication, such as perforation and peritonitis. Shoulder-top pain is an important symptom in patients with diffuse peritonitis.

At least 50% of all patients with cord injury have incomplete lesions. Allowance must be made for the faculties that may be distorted or lost because of the lesion. With careful attention to the symptoms and signs that are possible because of intact pathways early detection of abdominal disease and prompt treatment are possible.

REFERENCES

1. Apley J: The child with Abdominal Pains, 2d ed. Oxford: Blackwell, 1975.
2. Campbell IW, Duncan LJP, Innes JA, MacCuish AC, Munro JF: Abdominal pain in diabetic metabolic decompensation. JAMA 233:166–168, 1975.
3. Charney KJ, Juler GL, Comarr AE: General surgery problems in patients with spinal cord injuries. Arch Surg 110:1083–1088, 1975.
4. Cooperman EM: The child with recurrent abdominal pain. Can Med Assoc J 115:973–974, 1976.
5. Dodge JA: Recurrent abdominal pain in children. Br Med J 1:385–387, 1976.
6. Farmer DA: Abdominal pain. Med Clin North Amer 41:1287–1302, 1957.
7. Greenfield J: Abdominal operations on patients with chronic paraplegia. Arch Surg 59:1077–1087, 1949.
8. Hoen TI, Cooper IS: Acute abdominal emergencies in paraplegics. Am J Surg 75:19–24, 1948.
9. Ingberg HO, Prust FW: The diagnosis of abdominal emergencies in patients with spinal cord lesions. Arch Phys Med 49:343–348, 1968.
10. Stein JA, Tschudy DP: Acute intermittent porphyria. Medicine 49:1–16, 1970.
11. Steinheber FU: Medical conditions mimicking the acute surgical abdomen. Med Clin North Amer 57:1559–1567, 1973.

FURTHER READING

Cope Z: The Early Diagnosis of the Acute Abdomen, 14th ed. London: Oxford, 1972.

Harvey AM, Bordley J: Differential Diagnosis, 2d ed. Philadelphia: Saunders, 1972.

Gelin L, Nyhus LM, Condon RE: Abdominal Pain. Philadelphia: Lippincott, 1969.

Jones PF: Emergency Abdominal Surgery in Infancy, Childhood and Adult Life. Oxford: Blackwell, 1974.

Mellinkoff SM: The Differential Diagnosis of Abdominal Pain. New York: McGraw-Hill, 1957.

Passmore R, Robson JS: A Companion to Medical Studies. Oxford: Blackwell, 1974.

Shepherd JA: A Concise Surgery of the Acute Abdomen. Edinburgh: Churchill, Livingstone, 1975.

Shepherd JA: Surgery of the Acute Abdomen. Edinburgh: Livingstone, 1968.

Chapter 10

Principles of Managing Abdominal Pain

The cause of acute abdominal pain must be diagnosed without delay. Only with early accurate diagnosis is it possible to manage these patients correctly. In every case, soon after resuscitation is begun, a decision has to be made for laparotomy or close observation. Every physician responsible for care of patients must be able to recognize shock and hemorrhage, intraperitoneal perforation, acute peritonitis, bowel obstruction, bowel strangulation, and paralytic ileus. Almost all urgent surgical emergencies fall into one or more of these categories (Figure 20).

REACTION TO SEVERE STRESS

All patients who have serious abdominal pain are under severe stress. Remember the reactions to stress whether the result of disease or injury and provide supportive treatment. The reaction to severe stress may begin with catecholamine release causing vasoconstriction and selective redistribution of the circulation. This reaction is more evident with severe blood loss than with other severe stresses. Blood is diverted from the skin, muscles, gut, and kidneys to maintain

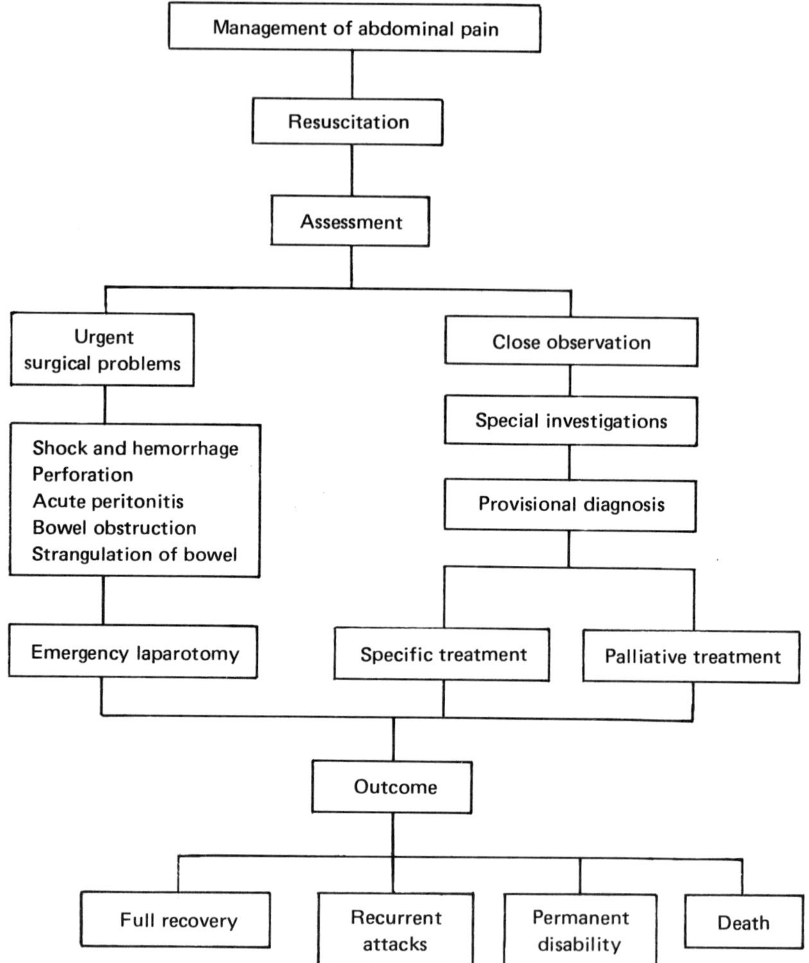

Figure 20 An outline of abdominal pain management and outcomes.

the circulation to the myocardium, lungs, and brain. Vascular refilling takes place by shift of fluids from interstitial tissues to the circulation in the early stages, and later fluids move out of the body cells (10). Falling blood pressure signals failure of compensation for hypovolemia.

The second phase of hypovolemic shock caused by hemorrhage or other major stress is characterized by fluid and sodium retention. A drop in renal artery pressure leads to decreased urine output, renin stimulated aldosterone secretion, further vasoconstriction by angiotensin II, and water and salt retention. The fluid is retained in the extravascular spaces causing hypoxia from pulmonary edema, confusion from cerebral edema, wound edema, edema at the site of the disease or injury, and diffuse edema throughout the body. In this phase the main management is myocardial, ventilatory, and renal support as needed.

Third phase is the mobilization of fluids that were sequestered in the second phase. There may be a temporary hypervolemia and elderly patients may develop congestive heart failure. The extra weight gain in the second phase is lost. Additional weight loss may be the first sign of body tissue breakdown, especially protein catabolism which is part of the reaction to injury.

Recovery is the last phase and it includes the reversal of catabolism and anabolic repair of body tissues during convalescence. To summarize the systemic reactions to severe stress:

First phase: Redistribution of circulation; hypoperfusion of skin, muscles, gut, kidneys; maintained perfusion of lungs, heart, brain

Second phase: Sodium and water conservation

Third phase: Mobilization of sequestered fluid, body tissue catabolism

Fourth phase: Repair of body tissues

URGENT ABDOMINAL PAIN PROBLEMS

Management of urgent abdominal pain problems always begins with resuscitation and immediate assessment. This immediate assessment separates those patients requiring urgent surgical care from those who may be kept under close observation following resuscitation.

Resuscitation is needed for all patients who have been injured or who have developed a serious illness rapidly. The essential measures in the initial management of a patient in hypovolemic shock are (2):

Make certain airway is clear and ventilation is adequate.

Stop external bleeding and examine for internal bleeding.

Insert a large central venous catheter, take blood for typing and matching, give saline rapidly intravenously, give blood when available as needed.

Insert urinary catheter and record hourly urine output.

Insert nasogastric tube, continuous gastric suction.

Anticipate hypoxia: give oxygen.

Watch all vital signs including general condition, state of consciousness, pulse, blood pressure, respiration, urine volume, central venous pressure, electrocardiogram, arterial blood gases, serum electrolytes.

Anticipate multiple blood transfusions: for acidosis give sodium bicarbonate, for hypocalcemia give calcium gluconate, for edema give plasma or albumin, for coagulation defect give fresh frozen plasma, avoid fibrillation by warming the blood during transfusion.

Treat any other complication such as anemia; respiratory, cardiac, or renal failure, or blood-clotting abnormality.

Shock and Hemorrhage

Shock and hemorrhage are recognized by tachycardia, falling blood pressure, poor skin circulation, prostration, and decreasing urinary flow. Hemorrhage is differentiated from the other causes of shock in the early stages by more prominent circulatory changes, pallor, thirst, air hunger, drowsiness, and a falling hematocrit. If the site of hemorrhage is not obvious, continue to re-examine the two large body cavities. Repeated chest X-rays are needed. Girth measurement of the abdomen may not be reliable unless air swallowing is managed by continuous gastric suction. Diagnostic peritoneal lavage is most helpful in recognizing intraperitoneal hemorrhage. Shock is always secondary; the cause must be found and treated.

Perforation

Perforation of a hollow viscus is characterized by the sudden onset of acute peritonitis with severe abdominal pain, which if not diffuse at first, rapidly becomes so. The site of the perforation is suggested by the place where the pain began. However, in a few cases perforation may be accompanied by temporary relief of pain as a distended viscus or abscess is suddenly decompressed by the perforation. If perforation occurs with sudden cessation of pain, the site of the pain prior to perforation indicates the location of the organ that ruptured. As a rule appendiceal, paracolic, and paracholecystic abscesses are readily diagnosed by an acutely painful tender mass complicating acute appendicitis, acute diverticulitis, or acute cholecystitis. When free perforation occurs, all such patients require resuscitation, peritoneal drainage, antibiotics if indicated, and more definitive treatment as follows.

Acute Appendicitis with Perforation

Acute appendicitis with perforation results in diffuse peritonitis and requires immediate appendectomy because the obstructing fecalith may dislodge allowing cecal contents to flood the peritoneal cavity. The treatment of early acute appendicitis is appendectomy. Sometimes removal of the appendix is considered too dangerous or difficult. In this case the abdomen is washed clear of purulent exudate and drainage is established. The appendix should be removed electively after three months. If a right lower quadrant mass is found with acute appendicitis, most surgeons will resuscitate and closely observe the patient. If the symptoms, the systemic signs of infection, and the regional signs of peritonitis improve, nonoperative management should be continued and the appendiceal mass should resolve. If there is no improvement, drainage is established or lavage is used to treat the peritonitis. In either case appendectomy is performed three months later.

Acute Diverticulitis with Free Perforation

Acute diverticulitis with free perforation results in diffuse peritonitis and requires immediate exploration to make certain that it is a purulent peritonitis rather than a wide perforation with fecal peritonitis. A purulent peritonitis requires peritoneal lavage and adequate drainage. Immediate resection or transverse colostomy may not be needed because purulent peritonitis from diverticulitis is infrequently followed by fecal peritonitis in the absence of distal obstruction. However, fecal peritonitis from colonic rupture must be treated by immediate resection. Exteriorization of the proximal and distal ends of the bowel is safest after resection, although the distal end may be closed and left in the pelvic cavity. A proximal colostomy should be used to provide protection from leakage if an anastomosis is performed following resection. The abdominal cavity must be drained; operative and postoperative lavage should be considered.

Acute Cholecystitis with Perforation and Acute Peritonitis

Acute cholecystitis with perforation and acute peritonitis requires immediate cholecystectomy because it is caused by gangrene of the gallbladder wall and continuing bile leakage should be anticipated. In a poor risk patient cholecytostomy and, if needed because of leakage, drainage or lavage of the peritoneal cavity can be carried out under local anesthesia (3). Paracholecystic abscess is a more frequent complication than perforation of the gallbladder with diffuse peritonitis.

Duodenal Ulcer with Perforation

Duodenal ulcer with perforation causes widespread, sudden onset, steady abdominal pain with signs of diffuse severe peritonitis. It is best treated by immediate laparotomy and closure of the perforated ulcer and possibly an ulcer operation if conditions are suitable.

Perforation of Strangulated or Obstructed Intestine

Perforation of strangulated or obstructed intestine occurs through a patch of gangrene so that lavage, resection of bowel, and drainage are necessary. Similarly perforations of bowel caused by typhoid or tuberculous or amoebic infection also require resection after thorough aspiration and peritoneal lavage.

Perforated Toxic Megacolon

Perforated toxic megacolon is a serious complication requiring resection of the colon and ileostomy. The usual causes are ulcerative colitis and Crohn's disease of the colon. The rectum is removed at the same time or later if deemed safer. Unperforated toxic megacolon may require resection or decompression and ileostomy.

Acute Peritonitis

The cardinal sign of acute peritonitis is involuntary muscle guarding. Useful but less reliable signs are remote rebound and percussion tenderness and hyperesthesia. Soon after peritonitis develops, paralytic ileus occurs so that bowel sounds are lost, no gas or feces are passed by rectum, vomiting may occur, and the abdomen may enlarge especially if there is no nasogastric suction. It is very important to be able to recognize involuntary muscle guarding. There are only a few rare causes of involuntary muscle guarding apart from peritoneal irritation. These are spasticity resulting from spinal cord injury or disease, heat stroke, adrenal crisis, hyperparathyroidism with hypercalcemia, and black widow spider bite. In these cases there is no deep tenderness although the abdominal wall muscles may be tender from sustained contraction.

Primary peritonitis is very rare. Always assume peritonitis is secondary and search for a cause. Most inflammatory lesions causing acute peritonitis are associated with fever, leukocytosis, and general malaise. Peritoneal irritation is also caused by intraperitoneal blood, bile, bowel contents, and infected urine. There is diffuse tenderness with diffuse peritonitis. If tenderness is more severe in one region, search for the cause of peritonitis there. There is direct tenderness over the inflamed ruptured viscus and often remote tenderness in other parts of the abdomen. Local percussion tenderness, local rebound tenderness, and remote rebound tenderness are almost always present with acute peritonitis.

Other than resuscitation, drainage, and possibly antibiotics, the treatment of acute peritonitis depends upon the cause. Almost all causes require surgical management, and the majority need urgent laparotomy.

Mechanical Bowel Obstruction

Mechanical bowel obstruction is characterized by intestinal cramps, hyperactive bowel sounds, no gas or feces passed by rectum, abdominal distension, and nausea and vomiting. All patients require resuscitation. Gastrointestinal decompression by nasogastric suction is always necessary; colonic decompression by cleansing enemas should be used providing there is no sign of peritoneal irritation and therefore no sign of bowel perforation. With time the abdominal cramps may disappear; a steady pain remains as the obstructed bowel fatigues and dilates. If fever, tachycardia, leukocytosis, tenderness, or guarding develop, strangulation must be suspected. All patients with complete mechanical bowel obstruction require emergency operation soon after resuscitation is begun to avoid the much higher risk of perforation or strangulation of bowel.

Incomplete bowel obstruction is characterized by intestinal cramps, hyperactive bowel sounds, abdominal distension, possibly nausea and vomiting, and diarrhea more frequently than obstipation. With some cases of incomplete obstruction as with all cases of complete mechanical bowel obstruction early operation is needed because of the severity of the attack or the condition of the patient. However, the majority of patients with incomplete or recurrent bowel obstruction are given resuscitation and supportive measures, including decompression of the gastrointestinal tract, and are kept under close observation for a short trial of nonoperative treatment. If there are no signs of relief of the obstruction within an hour or two, laparotomy is indicated.

Strangulation of Bowel

Strangulation complicates mechanical bowel obstruction especially if caused by irreducible hernia, volvulus, or other closed-loop obstruction or if treatment of mechanical obstruction is delayed. In these cases the symptoms and signs of mechanical obstruction become severe and change as strangulation begins. Cramps become less evident as steady pain increases. Abdominal tenderness, both direct and remote; rebound tenderness, both direct and remote; percussion tenderness; and muscle guarding appear. The pulse quickens and weakens, and hypotension and prostration occur with the onset of shock. Local tenderness, muscle guarding, and tachycardia must be considered signs of strangulation when they appear in a patient with bowel obstruction.

Early surgical release of uncomplicated bowel obstruction is the only method of avoiding the high risk inherent in resecting obstructed bowel. With signs of early bowel strangulation immediate surgical resection is the only method of avoiding the very high risk inherent in treating bowel obstruction complicated by perforation. Because of the frequency and danger of early strangulation and perforation of closed-loop obstructions, this type of obstruction should be considered in every case of complete bowel obstruction.

Strangulation of the bowel may be primary rather than secondary to mechanical obstruction. The venous drainage or arterial supply may be blocked by thrombus or embolus, external pressure from tumor mass, mesenteric hemorrhage, or decreased flow in the splanchnic circulation. Both embolism and thrombosis may cause abrupt onset of abdominal pain; however, with thrombosis the onset may be more gradual. Rapid reduction of circulation to the bowel causes sudden, severe spasm and severe visceral pain, followed by a large secretion of mucus, water, or blood into the lumen causing fluid bowel movements. The submucosa of the ischemic bowel is swollen by edema and hemorrhage. Paralytic ileus ensues despite diarrhea. There are local signs of tenderness and peritoneal irritation and general signs of shock. Plain radiographs of the abdomen may show paralytic ileus and thickening of the bowel wall involved. Selective arteriograms may demonstrate the block but this is useful only in the earliest stages while there is still time to relieve an arterial block and restore the circulation and the bowel to normal.

If the diagnosis is made too late for successful embolectomy, thrombectomy, or by-pass graft, the patient is resuscitated and closely observed. If the pain, the systemic signs of shock, and the regional signs of peritonitis do not improve within an hour or so, laparotomy is required for resection of gangrenous bowel, bowel anastomosis or colostomy, and peritoneal drainage or lavage. If the symptoms, the signs of systemic shock, and the regional signs of peritonitis improve, nonoperative management may be continued on the assumption that the necrosis of the bowel is incomplete or the gangrenous segment is being successfully walled off from the peritoneal cavity. This allows time for full resuscitation and better preparation for delayed operation. A proximal colostomy is used for ischemia of distal colon. Eventually resection of the necrotic or stenotic bowel and restoration of bowel continuity becomes necessary.

Paralytic Ileus

Paralytic ileus is the result of one of many discoverable causes. Treacherous causes, such as intraperitoneal hemorrhage, bowel perforation, or bowel strangulation, may be present, and signs of peritoneal irritation are sometimes deceptively mild or absent. Indeed, paralytic ileus may be the only sign of serious peritonitis.

In postoperative patients the disappearance of bowel sounds after they have once returned following operation is a very important sign. In a postoperative patient this is frequently the only early abdominal sign of anastomosis leakage. Postoperative shock with paralytic ileus may be due to gangrene or perforation of bowel, septicemia or septic shock, or severe intraperitoneal hemorrhage; all are serious surgical emergencies.

MANAGEMENT BY CLOSE OBSERVATION

All patients with acute abdominal pain problems are resuscitated and assessed. Patients with urgent surgical problems are identified for immediate operation. If there is no clear evidence of an urgent surgical complication, patients may be kept under close observation following resuscitation. These patients are closely watched for delayed appearance of symptoms and signs of a serious complication because some of these patients may have acute appendicitis or another problem that requires early operation. Others may undergo further investigation for diagnosis.

If close observation is the management chosen, some types of patients may show deceptively mild responses to serious disease. Be especially watchful of the very young; the very old; the malnourished; the very obese; patients on adrenocorticosteroids or immunosuppressive drugs, with widespread malignant disease or decreased levels of consciousness, in renal or hepatic failure, in the early postoperative period; paraplegics and quadriplegics; women in late pregnancy. Severe abdominal pain lasting six hours or longer is likely to be caused by a condition requiring surgical operation (1). Close observation is safe only when conducted by a clinician fully aware of the clinical characteristics of urgent surgical complications.

CHRONIC PAIN

A chronic pain problem is assumed to result from an undiagnosed or untreatable cause. Chronic pain might be caused by malignant tumor, painful phantom limb, causalgia, sympathetic dystrophy, herpes zoster, or idiopathic inflammatory process. Once it is realized that the cause is untreatable, attention should be given to all possible methods of obtaining relief. A number of disciplines may be involved in deciding the best treatment; this is the justification for pain clinics (8). For example, the patient may be a candidate for laparotomy for celiac ganglionectomy by a general surgeon, a cervical cordotomy by a neurosurgeon, or phenol instillation into the subarachnoid space by lumbar puncture by an anesthesiologist.

Chronic pain may remain undiagnosed for a long period of time. As a rule steady pain lasting six months or longer without relief is the result of unrecognized malignant tumor or is psychogenic. In malignant disease chronic pain usually grows worse and eventually the malignancy declares itself by the appearance of a mass, complications, or significant deterioration in the patient's health.

Psychogenic pain may torment the unfortunate individual continuously for an indefinite period of time, often with little change in the patient's health. The management of patients with psychogenic pain is not directed toward relief of pain but toward finding the reason for the patient's complaint. Once the reason for complaining is identified, a number of treatments might be used, such as group therapy, supportive therapy, and assistance through social agencies. If a patient having psychogenic pain is concentrating on one particular organ system, sometimes that system must be thoroughly investigated to releive the patient's anxiety, especially with cancerophobia. Only after negative investigations may these patients accept reassurance that there is no evidence of malignant disease. However frankly neurotic patients simply switch their attention to another set of complaints.

Some patients with psychogenic pain insist that they are seriously ill with persisting, acute pain. Their physicians may become anxious and frustrated as investigations reveal no abnormality and there is no response to therapy, including analgesics. Once psychogenic pain is recognized, the self-diagnosis of acute pain should be denied; yet continuing care should be offered for chronic pain (4). During management of the underlying emotional problem, secondary disorders, such as drug dependency, should be treated.

No matter what the cause of their complaints, some patients are particularly difficult to manage. They may use denial or rejection in order to manipulate helpers, or they may become helpless or demanding in order to receive additional attention. These individuals tax their physicians' patience, judgment, and emotional control and may evoke feelings of aversion, anxiety, depression, guilt, or even malice (6). Patients having these characteristics should be recognized early so that appropriate methods of managing their behavior can be applied while providing medical care for their complaints. The methods are described in Chapter 1.

DIAGNOSTIC DIFFICULTIES

What can be done when it appears to be impossible to make a diagnosis; yet the physician is convinced that the patient is in pain? Psychogenic pain will have been considered if there are exaggerations; inconsistencies; inappropriate complaints or behavior; symptoms incompatible with anatomical, physiological, or medical facts; unusual developments; or multiple irrelevant complaints. Similarly if there are multiple symptoms in a number of organ systems, particularly high fever, chills or rigors, profuse diarrhea, pain and stiffness in joints, and skin eruptions systemic disease will have been considered.

It will remain eternally true that full history and complete physical examination are the first steps in clinical diagnosis. If a reasonable hypothesis can be formulated, appropriate investigation will lead to rational managment. If the problem remains obscure and there is no clear path to follow, three options are available. The first option is to ask for a consultation; no physician who is truly interested in helping patients would hesitate to seek help from another clinician (Figure 21).

Sometimes the wisest move is to make a provisional diagnosis and prescribe what appears to be the most appropriate treatment. This is a trial where the effects of treatment are closely watched; success supports the diagnosis. A patient might be placed on an ulcer regimen on the basis of symptoms alone. Control of symptoms and prevention of recurrences are signs of successful treatment that support the provisional diagnosis but do not confirm it because, in this example, patients having reflux esophagitis or gastritis would also improve from this treatment. The treatment is appropriate, but the diagnosis might be incorrect.

Sometimes the best choice when in difficulty is close observation. Provided that inactivity is safe, close observation will often allow further evolution of the disease to be studied. The patient may recover, and a firm diagnosis may not be made. If recovery does not take place, changes will be observed eventually that will lead to an understanding of the disease. A patient having right lower abdominal pain without tenderness or peritoneal irritation could be watched with safety while awaiting resolution or more positive signs of appendicitis.

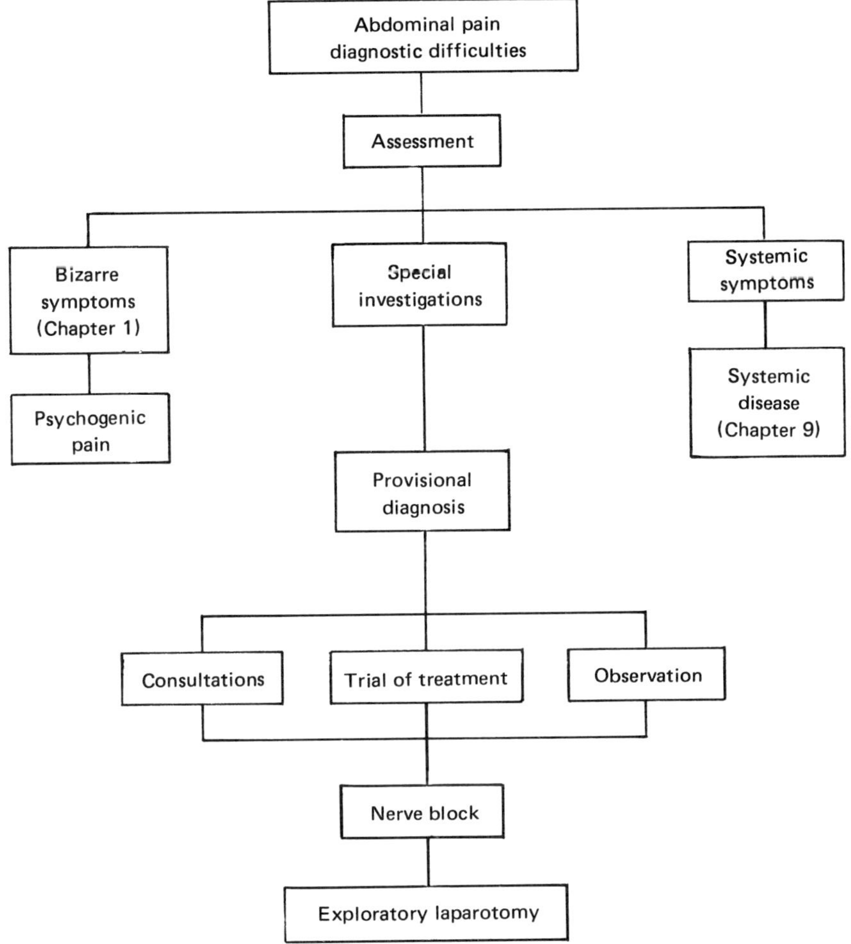

Figure 21 A plan for managing abdominal pain when there is great difficulty in making a diagnosis.

When patients complain of distress described as severe, crampy pain, the likelihood that the pain is from smooth muscle contraction is accurately tested by giving an injection of a potent nonanalgesic antispasmodic, such as atropine, provided that there are no contraindications, such as glaucoma or prostatism. An adequate dose of the antispasmodic arrests smooth muscle spasm and confirms that spasm is the cause of the pain. There is no benefit if the pain derives from another mechanism.

If the emotional reaction to pain seems disproportionate, give an injection of a sedative or tranquilizer with little analgesic effect. Do not be misled by the patient's feeling better because even patients in severe pain feel somewhat better with partial relief from distress caused by fear and anxiety.

Nerve Blocks

When pain seems confined to a limited area, especially to one dermatome, it is practical to consider a nerve block. Interpret the results carefully. Benefit might be gained from sensory nerve block, local vasodilatation, motor nerve block relieving skeletal muscle contractions, or numbing of a nerve that has become painful because of local pressure or other phenomena. In other words real improvement in the pain following a nerve block confirms the source of the pain but not the mechanism.

The sensitivity of nerves to local anesthetic agents is related to the size of the fiber and the duration of exposure (5). This fact is used in differential epidural or spinal nerve blocks. A patient having a perplexing pain problem is given initially a spinal or epidural placebo injection of saline. After this effect is studied it may be followed by injection of a dilute solution of a local anesthetic agent. If there is no sensory deficit, any benefit from the injection is assumed to be caused by anesthesia of narrow fibers only. A medium concentration of local anesthetic agent can be given, and relief suggests that the pain is carried by wide sensory fibers. If relief of the pain does not follow the injection of a concentrated solution of the local anesthetic agent, either there is a central mechanism or the patient is a malingerer (14).

Exploratory Laparotomy

When patients have persisting abdominal pain, yet all attempts to find the cause have failed, an exploratory laparotomy may be suggested. Laparotomy provides an opportunity for a complete physical examination of the viscera of the abdomen and pelvis. The only abdominal organs difficult to assess at laparotomy are the kidneys so that a preoperative intravenous pyelogram is a necessity.

Surgical operation should not be considered unless medical causes of abdominal pain have been eliminated, such as uncontrolled diabetes mellitus, acute hepatitis, or acute pancreatitis. Because laparotomy may be harmful, it is not needed for diagnosis in such cases unless one feels that two diseases are present. The highest incidence of unnecessary laparotomy lies in young women. The greatest danger of harm from laparotomy is in older men, but the yield is highest. In cases of upper abdominal pain myocardial infarction, acute hepatitis, pulmonary embolus, and pneumonia must be ruled out by appropriate investigation. When cholecystitis because of gallstones is suspected but ruled out by X-ray investigations, examine for renal disease, pancreatitis, or hepatitis as possible causes of right upper abdominal pain (7). Recommend exploratory laparatomy with caution because there is risk to the operation. With careful preoperative assessment the yield is low (12, 15). The chances of positive findings to explain abdominal pain vary according to the incidence of preoperative positive objective findings on physical examination, laboratory tests, and radiological investigations. When there are no preoperative positive findings in any of these categories, diagnosis at laparotomy will be unlikely (11).

Laparotomy without a reasonably firm diagnosis is wrong in almost all cases. Occasionally, well-meaning physicians and surgeons are misled by an arteriogram, isotopc scan, or ultrasound study into believing that disease is present. The patient may be subjected to one of a series of poorly indicated explorations. Every laparotomy carries with it the risk of anesthesia complications, wound infection, or peritoneal adhesions. Similarly, laparoscopy, which can be especially helpful in examination of the female pelvic organs, is not without risk.

When pain is the main problem before operation and laparotomy reveals an untreatable lesion, such as carcinoma of the pancreas with metastases, the surgeon should be prepared to interrupt pain pathways. In the case of carcinoma of the pancreas, for example, the surgeon should consider destruction of the visceral pain pathways by celiac ganglionectomy (13). Alternatively, if operation is otherwise not needed, these pathways may be destroyed by percutaneous celiac plexus block with alcohol under local anesthesia (19).

Treatment by placebo administration is not recommended, but a single injection of saline may have diagnostic value. When a placebo is effective in relieving pain, even though temporarily, it is assumed that the benefit is a result of mind over body (8). Placebos must be used cautiously to prevent the patient from realizing that he or she has been tricked, thus destroying trust in the physician. Surgical operations can have a placebo effect. Many exploratory laparotomies and other operations of no possible benefit other than to please the patient or the surgeon have brought about temporary relief, but this relief rarely lasts more than three months.

Safe management of patients with abdominal pain presents a major challenge. The knowledge and techniques necessary for correct clinical assessment are not complicated. The symptoms and signs of urgent surgical complications are clear in most cases. Early, correct management provides the best chance of avoiding much morbidity and possible mortality. The responsibility for accurate diagnosis and safe management rests in the hands of every practitioner who cares for patients with abdominal pain.

REFERENCES

1. Cope Z: The Early Diagnosis of the Acute Abdomen, 14th ed. London: Oxford, 1972.

2. Currie DJ: Early management of the critically injured. Can Med Assoc J 95:862–870, 1966.
3. Currie DJ: Continuous peritoneal lavage. Surg Gynecol Obstet 135:951–952, 1972.
4. DeVaul RA, Faillace LA: Persistent pain and illness insistence. Am J Surg 135:828–833, 1978.
5. Gasser HS, Erlanger J: The role of fiber size in the establishment of a nerve block by pressure or cocaine. Am J Physiol 88:581–590, 1929.
6. Groves JE: Taking care of the hateful patient. N Engl J Med 298:883–887, 1978.
7. Halasz NA: Counterfeit cholecystitis. Am J Surg 130:189–193, 1975.
8. Hannington-Kiff JG: Pain Relief. Philadelphia: Lippincott, 1974.
9. Jones J, Gough D: Celiac plexus block with alcohol for relief of upper abdominal pain due to cancer. Ann R Coll Surg Engl 59:46–49, 1977.
10. Lucas CE: Resuscitation of the injured patient; the three phases of treatment. Surg Clin North Am 57:3–15, 1977.
11. Piedrahita P, Butterfield WC: Abdominal exploration as a diagnostic procedure. Am J Surg 131:181–184, 1976.
12. Sarfeh IJ: Abdominal pain of unknown etiology. Am J Surg 132:22–25, 1976.
13. White TT: Visceral pain. Postgrad Med J 53:199–202, 1973.
14. Winnie AP, Collins VJL: Pain clinic 1: Differential neural blockade in pain syndromes of questionable etiology. Med Clin North Am 52:123–129, 1968.
15. Yajko RD, Steele G: Exploratory celiotomy for acute abdominal pain. Am J Surg 128:773–776, 1974.

FURTHER READING

Currie DJ: Urgent gastrointestinal operations upon patients whose wounds heal poorly. Surg Gynecol Obstet 147:913, 1978.

Hinchey EJ, Schaal PGH, Richards GK: Treatment of perforated diverticular disease of the colon. In: Advances in Surgery, edited by C Rob. Chicago: Year Book, 1978, pp. 85–109.

Hunt JA, Rivlin ME, Clarebout HJ: Antibiotic peritoneal lavage in severe peritoneal lavage in severe peritonitis. S Afr Med J 49:233–238, 1975.

Passmore R, Robson JS: A Companion to Medical Studies. Oxford: Blackwell, 1974.

Taylor JD, Moore KA: Generalized peritonitis complicating diverticulitis of the sigmoid colon. J R Coll Surg Edin 21:348–352, 1976.

Index